Fractures of the Tibial Pilon

Springer

Milano
Berlin
Heidelberg
New York
Hong Kong
London
Paris
Tokyo

P. Bartolozzi • F. Lavini

Fractures of the Tibial Pilon

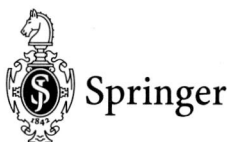 Springer

P. Bartolozzi
F. Lavini
Clinica Ortopedica e Traumatologica
Policlinico G.B. Rossi
Verona

Translation from the Italian Language edition
Le fratture del pilone tibiale by P. Bartolozzi and F. Lavini (eds)
© Springer-Velag Italia, Milan 2002

Translator: Logos Group, Modena, Italy
Final editing of the English edition: J.C.R. Scott, Orthofix, London

Springer-Verlag is a part of Springer Science+Business Media

© Springer-Verlag Italia, Milan 2004

ISBN 88-470-0248-6

Library of Congress Cataloging-in-Publication Data

Bartolozzi, P. (Pietro)
    [Fratture del pilone tibiale. English]
    Fractures of the tibial pilon / P. Bartolozzi, F. Lavini.
       p. cm.
    Includes bibliographical references.
    ISBN 8847002486 (alk. paper)
       1. Tibia--Fractures. I. Lavini, F. (Franco), 1959- II. Title.

    RD560.B3713 2004
    617.1'58--dc22

                                                            2004045251

Cover design: Simona Colombo, Milan, Italy
Typesetting: Graphostudio, Milan, Italy
Printing and binding: Signum, Bollate, Milan, Italy

Introduction

Pilon fractures represent 11% of all tibial fractures and are frequently caused by high energy trauma in young patients. The treatment can, therefore, be complex and the results disabling.

For this reason, the responsible surgeon must have a good understanding of the relevant anatomy and physiology and a thorough diagnostic examination protocol, which includes all the required images for a rational treatment approach to these lesions.

The therapeutic choice will be based upon many factors, such as the age of the patient, type of trauma and associated pathological conditions, including the vascularisation of the distal third of the tibia. The objectives are: accurate reconstruction of the joint, stability in order to allow early rehabilitation and reduce the frequently reported complications to a minimum.

Disabling results, such as stiffness or early arthrosis, are common since the injury can cause severe damage to the articular cartilage. For this reason, the methods of preventing these complications and post-traumatic reconstruction strategies are becoming of more interest. The variation of medical opinion, the details of the different treatment strategies and the modern possibilities for reconstructive surgery are particularly suitable for discussion in an instructional course for orthopaedic surgeons.

P. Bartolozzi
F. Lavini

Contents

An Overview of Tibial Pilon Fractures

Epidemiology and Pathological Anatomy

V. Caiaffa, D. De Vita, M. Di Viesto, G. Solarino Jr

With the growing number of road traffic accidents and high-energy trauma events over recent years, traumatology departments have seen an increasing incidence of complex bone injuries with comminuted fractures and extensive soft tissue damage; these include fractures of the distal tibial metaphysis, more commonly known as "tibial pilon" fractures.

The term "tibial pilon" was first used in 1911 by Destot who likened the shape of the distal tibia to a mortar and compared the explosive impact of the talus against the tibia to the action of a pestle against a mortar, similar to a hammer striking a nail [1].

In 1950 Bonin, when describing the distal metaphysis as the vault of ankle articulation, identified this type of injury with the term "fracture of the articular roof" ("plafond fracture"), and emphasised the frequent involvement of articular surfaces and therefore articular cartilage with all the related consequences [2-4].

Generally speaking, injuries of this type are relatively rare and account for 7-10% of fractured tibiae and less than 1% of fractures of the lower limbs [3, 5, 6], but they are increasing in number in line with road traffic accidents. About one half of these fractures are attributed to road traffic accidents (45.5%), followed by falls from a height (27.3%) [7]. They should be distinguished from the more common, low energy malleolar fractures, which are the result of rotational or angular forces that are not transmitted into the metaphysis.

Considering the violence of the forces at work, it is not surprising that these injuries are often associated with serious systemic problems in polytraumatised patients [8].

From the epidemiological point of view, tibial pilon injuries account for 2.1% of all fractures of the long bones. Males tend to suffer this type of injury slightly more than females with a peak incidence rate at about 45 years of age.

I Clinica Ortopedica, Università degli Studi di Bari

Because of their serious nature and the gravity of accompanying complications, these fractures are a very important element of the traumatologist's workload.

An overview of the distal tibial metaphysis with regard to anatomy and physiology will assist in providing a clearer understanding of the potential problems associated with these types of injuries.

The tibia widens distally into the metaphysis and extends medially into the medial malleolus. It has five surfaces: anterior, medial, posterior, lateral and inferior [9].

The *anterior surface* projects above the inferior surface, from which it is separated by a shallow groove, and merges proximally with the lateral surface of the diaphysis. The *medial surface* extends proximally into the antero-medial border of the diaphysis and distally into the medial surface of the malleolus.

The *posterior surface* is traversed at its medial extremity by, usually, a wide groove, which can be traced down to the posterior surface of the medial malleolus, and extends proximally into the posterior border of the diaphysis.

The *lateral surface* corresponds to the triangular fibular notch which is connected by ligaments to the inferior extremity of the fibula.

The *inferior surface* is smooth and articulates with the body of the talus. It is broader anteriorly, concave in the sagittal plane and slightly convex in the frontal plane. It is continuous with the articular surface of the medial malleolus [9].

Because of its anatomical shape, the profile of the distal tibia can be deceptive during fixator positioning. As a consequence nails, wires and screws can easily penetrate the joint. At least two orthogonal X-Rays should be taken to avoid such events occurring and ensure correct positioning of any fixator [10].

The medial malleolus is a short but sturdy process [9]. The medial face is an attachment for ligaments and is grooved to allow the passage of tendons for the flexor muscles. The lateral articular surface is flat in the sagittal plane and articulates with the medial aspect of the talar articular surface [11].

The ankle is a hinge joint and allows movement in one direction only. It regulates leg and foot movements in the sagittal plane, allowing flexion and extension movements around a transverse axis between the two malleoli [12].

The amount of possible plantar-flexion is greater than that of dorsi-flexion, with 20° of dorsi-flexion and 30° of plantar-flexion (or extension). Other types of movement within the tibio-talar joint are not permitted as the talus is firmly located within the tibio-fibular joint by a sturdy complex of ligaments. This joint can adjust in size thanks to the elasticity of the tibio-fibular joint to accommodate the varied width of the talus during articulation [12].

In mechanical terms, the tibio-tarsal joint can be described as follows:
- a lower part, the talus, offers an approximately cylindrical surface to the main transverse axis;
- an upper part, the distal extremities of the tibia and fibula, forms a block with a recessed lower face to locate the talar surface cylinder.

The complete cylinder mechanism is laterally fixed between the two sides of the upper part, which allows flexion and extension movements around a common axis [12].

In anatomical terms, the complete cylinder would be the talar pulley mechanism and the cylinder recess, the tibio-fibular mortar. The surface of the talar trochlea is convex looking from front to rear and slightly concave transversely; it is also wider at the rear than the front. The distal articulating surface of the tibia is exactly the opposite. The medial malleolus articulates with a small articular surface on the upper part of the medial talus; the lateral malleolus articulates with an articular surface on the lateral surface of the talus [12].

The joint is held together by a ligament-reinforced articular capsule. The fibrous section of the articular capsule is located on the margins of the tibio-fibular and talar articular surfaces [11].

Two main ligaments form the tibio-tarsal connection, the lateral and medial ligaments, which together support the mechanism. There are two additional systems: anterior and posterior ligaments which are simply capsular thickenings [12] and the side ligaments (lateral and medial) which form sturdy fibrous fans that are located on the corresponding malleolus on each side of the joint [12].

The range of flexion/extension movements is mainly governed by the degree to which the joint surfaces are developed. Given that the tibial surface can rotate to 70° and the talar trochlea to between 140°–150°, simple subtraction would therefore leave a flexion/extension range of between 70°–80°. It can also be seen that the pulley has more angular development forwards than backwards and this explains the greater degree of extension than flexion [12].

Anterior-posterior tibio-tarsal stability and contact between the joint elements are governed by gravity and retain the talus within the tibial surface area. The anterior and posterior edges of this surface form a ridge that stops the trochlea from sliding back and forth. The lateral and medial ligaments (and muscles) act as a retention system for the joint [12].

When flexion/extension movements go beyond their permitted limits, one of the elements of the joint must give way. Hyperextension can thus lead to either a posterior displacement or a fracture of the posterior edge.

Similarly forced dorsi-flexion can lead to an anterior displacement or a fracture of the anterior edge [12].

The tendons, blood vessels, and nerves anterior to the tibio-tarsal articulation are medio-laterally, tibialis anterior, extensor hallucis, anterior tibial vessels, deep peroneal nerve, extensor digitorum, and peroneus tertius, all held in position by the superior and inferior extensor retinaculi; posteriorly, from the medial side are tibialis posterior, the flexor digitorm longus, the posterior tibial vessels, the tibial nerve, and flexor hallucis longus; in the groove behind the fibular malleolus, the peroneal tendons are short and held in place by the superior and inferior retinaculi [9].

Blood is supplied to the tibio-tarsal joint by the malleolar branches of the tibial and fibular arteries. To maintain cutaneous blood supply when making incisions, a gap of 7-8 cm is recommended between tibial and fibular incisions [3]. Innervation is by branches of the deep peroneal and tibial nerves [9].

A particular characteristic of this anatomical region is the relative absence of muscle elements which has a negative effect on blood supply. The only muscle that covers the anterior surface of the distal tibia is extensor digitorum. The only muscle on the posterior surface is flexor hallucis. There is no other lateral or medial muscular cover.

The skin in this area is particularly thin with little underlying adipose tissue.

The most frequent cause of pilon fractures is a direct vertical force exerted by the talus on the tibial plafond [13]. The "compression" specifically damages the tibio-talar surface of the joint.

The severity of osteo-cartilaginous injuries is directly proportional to the amount of energy absorbed by the tibia [14].

Somewhat less frequently, the forces that determine these injuries are exerted in a rotational direction and the resulting comminution is less severe [13].

These two types of forces are often exerted together, especially in road traffic accidents, and result in comminution with significant interfragmentary separation [13].

The relatively poor blood supply and thin overlying skin further complicate the clinical situation and compromise both the short and long-term results. The causes of this type of fracture are most frequently associated with road traffic accidents (especially with motorcyclists who instinctively try to brake with their feet before impact) and falls from heights. Talar injuries happen less often through accidents at work or during sport [6, 7].

The injuries can be divided into two categories based on aetiology:
- low-energy trauma events;
- high-energy trauma events.

Low-energy trauma is mainly associated with rotational stresses exerted on the distal tibia, as happens in sports accidents, (especially skiing accidents) and with spiral fractures that extend from the inferior tibial diaphysis to the ankle joint (Fig. 1) [15].

High-energy trauma, which is more frequent, is associated with axial force with or without an angular or rotational element, as happens in falls from a height or road traffic accidents. The forces exerted determine the impact of the talus against the tibio-peroneal articular surface, depressing it and frequently causing comminution of the tibial metaphysis (Fig. 2) [15].

The part of the tibial articular surface most affected by the force of axial compression is determined by the position of the foot at the moment of impact, because this influences the position of the tibial plafond and thus the degree of displacement and comminution [3]. When the feet are plantar flexed, the compression forces are directed backwards, and when dorsiflexed, the compression forces are directed forwards. When the feet are in the neutral position and the forces are vertical, the entire articular surface can be shattered, resulting in

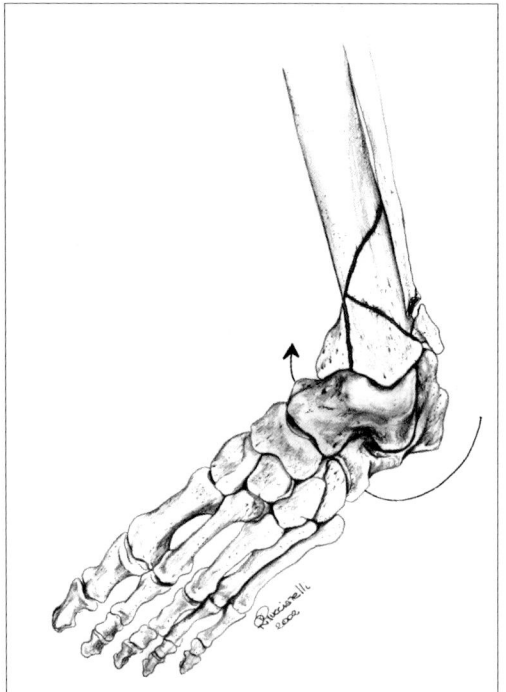

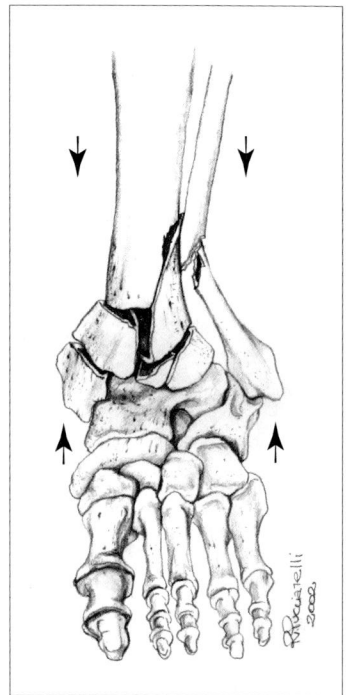

Fig. 1. Low-energy trauma, mainly rotational type injury

Fig. 2. High-energy trauma with axial effects

varying degrees of splintering of the metaphysis and compression of the joint surfaces [14].

In summary, a predominately rotational force generally results in large metaphyseal fragments with minimal compression and comminution of the joint. If axial compression is the direction of injury, it produces severe comminution of the joint with compressed fragments and involvement of the joint cartilage [10, 16].

The energy absorbed by the distal tibia during axial compression spreads to the soft tissues. This release of energy to an area unprotected by muscle, causes damage to the skin and subcutaneous tissue [17].

In 1984, Tscherne and Goetzen [18] classified injuries to the soft tissues associated with closed fractures, as shown in Table 1. The Authors stressed that the antero-medial section of the tibial distal metaphysis is at most risk. Unfortunately, this type of classification is not applicable to tibial pilon fractures given the lack of muscle cover.

Gustilo's 1984 classification [19] for open fractures is set out in Table 2.

In the presence of soft tissue injury, any surgical stabilisation operation should be as non-invasive as possible.

Table 1. Classification of soft tissue lesions according to Tscherne and Goetzen [17]

Grade 0:	Absence of soft tissue injuries
Grade I:	Abrasions or bruising to cutaneous and subcutaneous layers
Grade II:	Abrasions or bruising to the skin and near-surface muscles
Grade III:	Extended bruising with subcutaneous crushing and avulsion, severe injury to muscle tissue associated with compartmental syndrome and vascular lesions

Table 2. Gustilo and Anderson's classification of open fractures [15]

Type I:	Wound less than 2 cm long. No sign of contamination in the deep layers
Type II:	Wound more than 2 cm. No sign of severe load injury to the soft tissue
Type III:	High-energy impact. Large wound (greater than 10 cm) with severe soft tissue damage, in three categories
Type III A:	Large wound, but with potential for good soft tissue cover with local flaps
Type III B:	Large wound, and exposed bone fragments with extensive periosteal stripping. Skin cover is not possible without the use of remote flaps
Type III C:	Large wound with significant damage to the neurovascular supply

Regardless of the choice of surgical strategy, rapid intervention is recommended because of the high risk of bacterial proliferation when skin cover is lost. In these severe injuries oedema appears within 8-12 hours of the accident and remains for 8-10 days. All types of aggressive surgery should be avoided during this period [8].

In open fractures, thorough lavage and debridement together with external fixator fracture stabilisation are required. Soft tissue cover of open bones or joints should be achieved urgently along with fracture fixation [10, 20].

Blisters are indicators of soft tissue damage and may develop around the fracture after high-energy impact. These blisters may contain a clear or haemorrhagic fluid. They both indicate a tear in the dermal/epidermal layer, but those containing haemorrhagic fluid represent a more significant lesion from the histological and clinical point of view. It is very important not to incise such blisters, because this increases the risk of infection [10].

Oedema in taut and translucent skin contra-indicates "aggressive" surgery, as it may be impossible to close the incision and there is a risk of skin necrosis [20].

There have been various proposals for classifying these types of injuries. In 1953, Lauge-Hansen [21] proposed a classification based on the position of the feet at the moment of impact and on the direction of the force exerted on the tibio-fibulo-talar complex. He described pilon fractures as injuries associated with an accidental event causing forced pronation-dorsiflexion of the ankle/foot and as having four anatomo-pathological stages.

In 1979, Ruedi and Allgower proposed [22] an anatomical classification based on the degree of damage to the joint and comminution of the metaphysis. They subdivided the fractures into three types:
- Type I: articular fracture with minimal displacement;
- Type II: articular fracture with significant displacement without extensive comminution;
- Type III: articular fracture with significant joint displacement and comminution.

Also in 1979, Kellam and Waddell [15] proposed a classification system with two groups of fractures: A and B, defined according to the force that caused the injury, with a guide to prognosis.
- Type A fractures, resulting from *lower-energy* events, usually with a rotational element, with minimal anterior cortical tibial comminution and large-sized joint fragments. They are generally associated with a short oblique or transverse fibular fracture above the level of the vault, and usually have a better prognosis;
- Type B fractures, which are higher energy injuries with significant axial compression, usually producing severe anterior cortico-tibial comminution, multiple articular fragmentation and metaphyseal extension often not associated with a fibular fracture. The prognosis is significantly worse [15].

In 1986, Ovadia and Beals [23], still using morphological criteria, modified Ruedi and Allgower's anatomical classification into five groups, with the following criteria:
- Type I: non-displaced articular fractures;
- Type II: minimally displaced fractures;
- Type III: displaced fractures with a small number of large fragments;
- Type IV: articular fractures with displacement multiple fragments and metaphyseal extension;
- Type V: articular fractures with displacement, severe comminution and a metaphyseal defect.

Types I and II Ovadia and Beals fractures correspond with Ruedi and Allgower Type I, Ovadia and Beals Type III correspond with Type II Ruedi and Allgower, and Types IV and V Ovadia and Beals correspond with Ruedi and Allgower Type III.

The Ovadia and Beals classification system improved on that of Ruedi and Allgower thanks to the introduction of metaphyseal extension in pilon fractures with both comminution and serious metaphyseal defects. However, none of these classifications distinguishes *high-energy impact* events (usually the result of road traffic accidents) which include diaphyseal extension into the middle third of the tibia [23].

Currently, a commonly used system is the AO classification proposed by the Müller study group in 1987 [24], which defines the distal tibial metaphysis as an area inside a square whose lower side traces the profile of the articular surfaces, and divides the fractures into three groups (Fig. 3):

A: extra-articular;
B: partially involving the articular fracture-line;
C: complete.

Each group is further sub-divided into three groups indicating the degree of comminution and the direction of the fracture–line(s).

Open tibial pilon fractures most frequently belong to group C (72.7%) followed by group A (18.2%) and B (9.1%). Using the Gustilo classification system for open fractures there is an incidence of 18.2% for Type I, 9% for Type II, 45.4% for Type III A and 27.3% for Type III B.

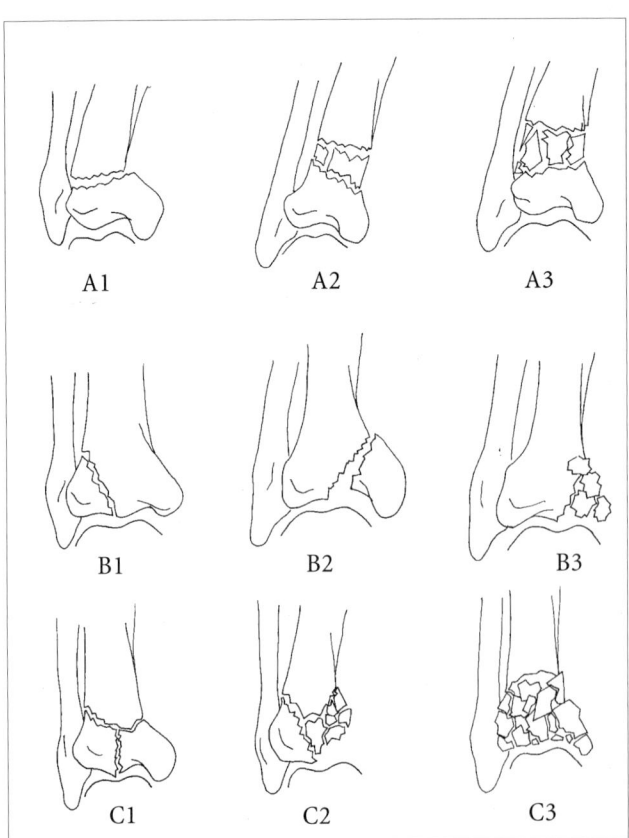

A1   A2   A3

B1   B2   B3

C1   C2   C3

Fig. 3. Classification AO tibial pilon fractures

The treatment of high-energy pilon fractures represents a real challenge to orthopaedic surgeons. Various treatment options have been used over time with disappointing, if not disheartening, results.

Most Authors would agree that the aim of treating these intra-articular displaced injuries should be to return the articular surface to normal and achieve stable synthesis that will allow early mobility of the joint and thus improved functional recovery.

References

1. Destot EAJ (1911) Traumatismes du pied et rayons X: malleoles-astragale-calcaneum-avant-pied. Masson, Paris
2. Bonin JG (1950) Injuries to the ankle. William Heinemann, London, pp 248-260
3. Helfet DL, Koval K, Pappas J et al (1994) Intra-articular "pilon" fracture of the tibia. Clin Orthop 298:221-228
4. Mc Donald MG, Burgess RC, Bolano LE, Nicholls PJ (1996) Ilizarov treatment of pilon fractures. Clin Orthop 325:232-238
5. Griffiths GP, Thordarson DB (1996) Tibial plafond fractures: limited internal fixation and a hybrid external fixator. Foot Ankle Int 17(8):444-448
6. Bourne RB (1989) Pilon fractures of the distal tibia. Clin Orthop 240:42-46
7. Court-Brown CM, Rimmer S, Prakash U, Mc Queen MM (1998) The epidemiology of open long bone fractures. Injury 29(7):529-534
8. Pierannunzii L, De Bellis U, d'Imporzano M (2002) Il trattamento chirurgico delle fratture del pilone tibiale. Giorn Ital Ortop Traumatol 28:11-23
9. Williams PL (1994) Anatomia del Gray, Italian edn. Zanichelli, Bologna
10. Thordarson DB (2000) Complications after treatment of tibial pilon fractures: prevention and management strategies. J Am Academy Orthop Surg 8(4):253-265
11. Balboni GC (1991) Anatomia umana. Ermes, Milano
12. Kapandji IA (1996) Fisiologia articolare, 4th edn. Monduzi, Paris
13. Mast JW, Spiegel PG, Pappas JN (1986) Fractures of tibial pilon. Clin Orthop 230:68-82
14. Rockwood CA Jr, Green DP (1996) Fractures in adults, Vol. 2, 4th edn. Lippincott-Raven, Philadelphia New York, pp 2236-2241
15. Kellam JF, Waddell JP (1979) Fractures of the distal metaphysis with intra-articular extension: the distal tibial explosion fracture. J Trauma 19(8):593-601
16. Leone VJ, Ruland R, Meinhard B (1993) The management of the soft tissues in pilon fractures. Clin Orthop 292:315-320
17. De Bastiani G, Graham Apley A, Goldberg A (2000) Orthofix external fixation in trauma and orthopaedics. Springer, Berlin Heidelberg New York
18. Tscherne H, Goetzen L (1984) Fractures with soft tissue injuries. Springer, Berlin Heidelberg New York
19. Gustilo RB, Mendoza RM, Williams DN (1984) Problems in the management of type III (severe) open fractures: a new classification of type III open fractures. J Trauma 24:742-746
20. Coughlin MJ, Mann RM (2001) Chirurgia del piede e della caviglia, Vol. 2, 7th edn. Verduci, Roma, pp 1346-1347
21. Lauge-Hansen N (1953) Fractures of the ankle: pronation-dorsiflexion fracture. Arch Surg 67:813

22. Ruedi TP, Allgower M (1979) The operative treatment of intra-articular fractures of the lower end of the tibia. Clin Orthop 138:105-110
23. Ovadia D, Beals RK (1986) Fractures of tibial plafond. J Bone Joint Surg Am 68(4):543-551
24. Müller ME, Allgower M, Schneider R, Willenegger H (1993) Manuale dell'osteosintesi: tecniche raccomandata dal gruppo AO, 3rd edn. Springer, Berlin Heidelberg New York

Anatomical and Radiological Classification of Pilon Tibial Fractures

C. Fialka, V. Vécsei

Introduction

Since the first description of tibial pilon fractures by Destot in 1911 [1] many Authors have attempted to describe the mechanism of this injury. The goal was to establish a classification system to help determine the prognosis and evaluate the clinical outcomes of these debilitating ankle fractures [2-10]. Pilon fractures account for 1 to 7% of all tibial fractures [11-14], and are accompanied by a variable degree of local soft tissue damage.

Several fracture classifications have demonstrated prognostic ability for the clinical outcome of pilon fractures [6-10]. Studies used to develop these classification systems have shown that the pathomorphology of the fracture, amount of comminution, displacement of fragments, and depression of the articular surface, are predictors of functional outcome. However, the influence of different treatment concepts on the clinical outcome of tibial pilon fractures is today still not clear, particularly as the degree of soft tissue damage is not also taken into consideration.

Historical Efforts and Fracture Mechanisms

The definition of a tibial pilon fracture is an intra-articular lesion of the distal metaphyseal component of the tibiae. The mechanism leading to this fracture type is mainly axial compression force, compressing the talar dome upwards into the distal tibial articular surface. Additional anterior or posterior shear forces due to the inclination of the hindfoot during injury may produce anterior and/or posterior fragments (see below).

University Hospital of Vienna, Medical School, Department of Traumatology, Vienna

Following descriptive case reports [15, 16], the first systematic classification was published by Böhler [2] who distinguished between extra-articular and intra-articular fractures. The intra-articular fractures were sub-classified according to the suspected fracture mechanisms (torsion, split forces, compression or bending forces etc.). The Böhler classification mainly concentrated on the split fragments and the anterior, posterior and medial components but did not refer to the central depressions, nor did it include metaphyseal comminution (Fig. 1). Based on Böhlers drawings, the classification by Gay and Evrard [4], later modified by Weber [17] and Ruedi et al. [5], was introduced in 1963. According to their study, which reviewed 241 cases, they concluded that capsular ruptures were responsible for fragment necrosis, but they also did not consider depression fractures of the articular surface.

Trojan and Jahna [3] emphasised the importance of restoring fibular length and recommended operative repair of the antero-lateral tibial fragment.

Weber [18] described in his monograph 3 types of intra-articular compression fractures of the distal tibia, dividing them into compression fractures of the tibia with:

1. fibula fractures with an intact syndesmosis,
2. additional talar fractures and
3. an intact fibula but syndesmotic rupture (Fig. 2).

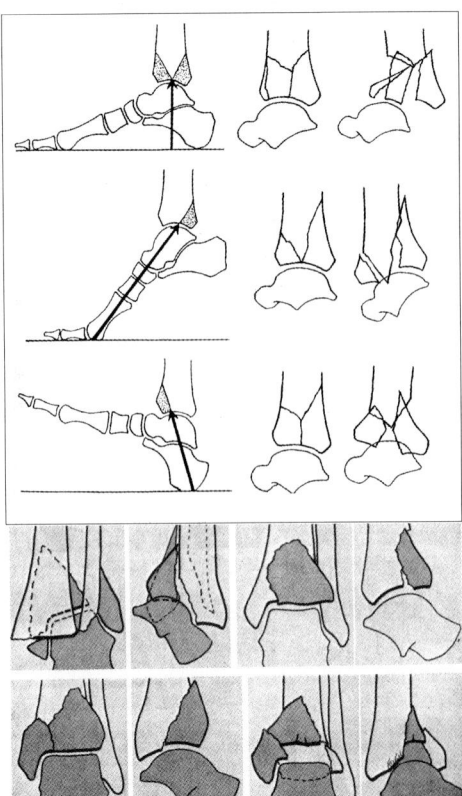

Fig. 1. Classification by Böhler (from [2] with permission). Schematic drawings from radiographs

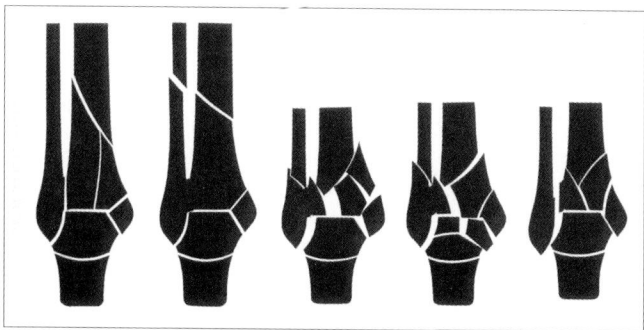

Fig. 2. Classification by Weber (from [18] with permission)

AO/ASIF Classification and Recent Developments

In the late 1960's Ruedi, Matter and Allgower [5] introduced a more detailed classification and added a therapeutic algorithm. The influence of the amount of displacement of the fragments, the degree of comminution, depression of the articular surface, defects in metaphyseal bone and concomitant fractures of the fibular are described. This work is the basis of the widely used AO/ASIF classification for this region (Fig. 3). In 1972 Heim published a paper that showed the importance of antero-lateral depressed fragments and the need for autologous cancellous bone graft in high energy comminuted fractures [19]. This has been supported by the findings of Vichard et al. [20] in 1973.

In 1978 Ruedi and Allgower [6] presented a modified classification, subclassifying the complete articular fractures into 3 types (Fig. 4):

-Type I: split fractures without dislocation;

-Type II: split fractures with significant dislocation;

-Type III: split fractures with significant dislocation and complex metaphyseal comminution.

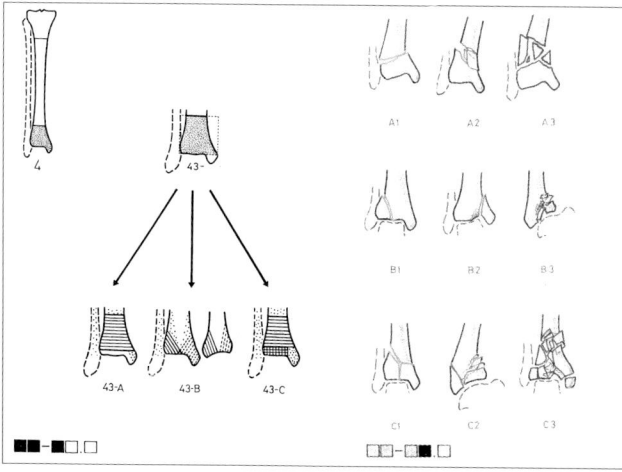

Fig. 3. AO/ASIF classification of the distal tibial segment ("43") (from [9] with permission)

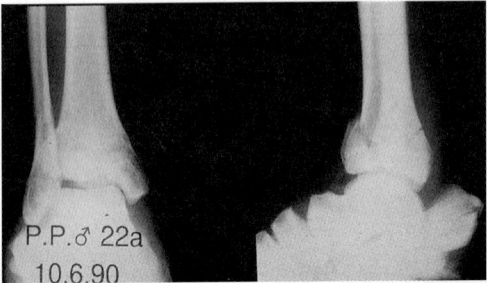

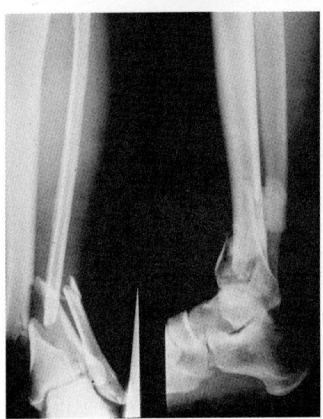
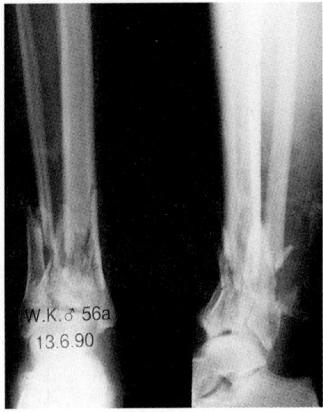

Fig. 4. Classification by Ruedi and Allgower (from [6] with permission) for the complete articular fracture ("43 C" according to AO/ASIF classification). **a** Type I: split fractures without dislocation. **b** Type II: split fractures with mark dislocation. **c** Type III: split fractures with mark dislocation and methapyseal comminution

Today's most commonly used classification is the "Comprehensive Classification of Fractures of Long Bones" first published by Müller [9]. As mentioned above, for the distal tibial segment the findings of Ruedi and Allgower are the fundamental basis for this classification (Fig. 5), which follows the AO documentation principles. Therefore the metaphyseal segment of the tibiae is classified as "43" and the fracture Types A (extra-articular), B (partial articular) and C (complete articular fractures) respectively. By definition tibial pilon fractures can only be rated as B or C. The subgroups give information about the mechanism of injury (split forces leading to B1 or C1 fractures; compression forces leading to various types of depressions, such as a simple depression in partial split fractures B2.1, or in complete split fractures C1.2 etc.).

Following the logical course of the AO/ASIF classification, the B1.1 must be considered the most simple tibial pilon fracture type, and the C3.3 the most severe. But more importantly, when it comes to different kinds of depressed fragment, this classification offers a valid guide for the choice of operative procedures. The necessity for additional cancellous bone grafting, the method of restoring the articular surface and other parameters can by derived from this classification.

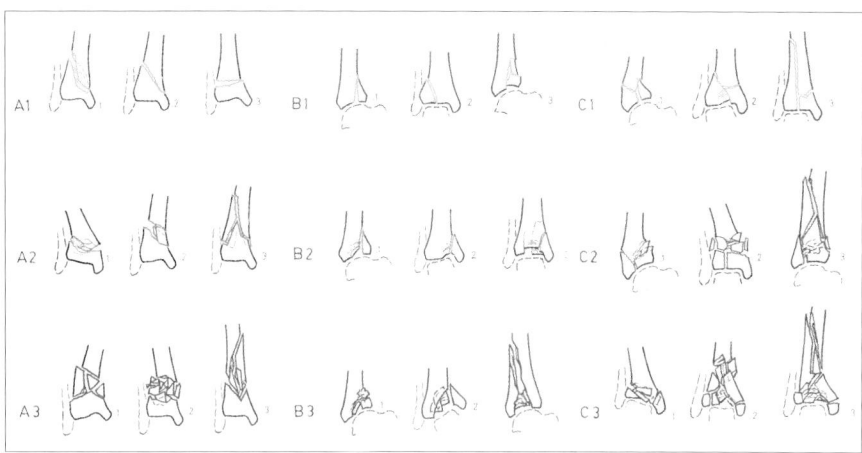

Fig. 5. *AO/ASIF classification by Müller* (from [9] with permission). *Classification for the intrarticular fractures of the distal tibial segment ("43").* **a** Extra-articular fractures. **b** Partial articular fractures; *B1.1:* simple split in lateral view; *B1.2:* simple split in ap view; *B1.3:* simple split on articular level, multiple metaphyseal split; *B2.1:* split with anterior impression; *B2.2:* split with medial or lateral impression; *B2.3:* split, central impression, metaphysis comminuted; *B3.1:* partial complex fracture of the articular surface, dorsal intact; *B3.2:* partial complex fracture of the articular surface lateral intact; *B3.3:* partial complex fracture of the articular surface, metaphysis comminuted. **c** Complete articular fractures; *C1.1:* articular split, simple metaphysis comminuted ("y-shaped"); *C1.2:* articular impression, simple metaphyseal component; *C1.3:* articular depression, complex metaphyseal component ("y-" or "t-shaped"); *C2.1:* articular split (depression possible), metaphyseal compression; *C2.2:* articular split and/or depression, metaphyseal comminution; *C2.3:* articular split and/or, metaphyseal and/or diaphyseal comminution; *C3.1:* comminuted articular and distal metaphysis; *C3.2:* comminuted articular and proximal metaphysis; *C3.3:* comminuted articular and distal diaphysis

In the following years various papers attempted to specify the importance of certain fragments in comminuted fractures, and derive a therapeutic prognosis out of these detailed findings.

However, as mentioned by Heim in his outstanding monograph about this topic [21], in the past few years the discussion in the literature has returned to a more general view of this problem. This has happened for two major reasons: the poor reproducibility of extremely detailed classifications in daily practice on a radiological bases, and the fact that a complex injury, involving multiple variations of bony and soft tissue injuries, is not solved by concentrating on the details of repair only.

References

1. Destot E (1911) Traumatisme du pied et rayons X. Masson, Paris
2. Böhler L (1951) Die Technik der Knochenbruchbehandlung. 12-13. Auflage, Maudrich Wien (Nachdruck 1977)
3. Trojan E, Jahna H (1956) Zur Behandlung der Stauchungsbrüche am distalen. Unterschenkelende Klin Med 11:313-317
4. Gay R, Evrard J (1963) Les fractures récentes du pilon tibial chez l'adult. Rev Chir Orthop 49: 397-512
5. Ruedi T, Matter P, Allgower M (1968) Die Intrartikulären Frakturen des distalen Unterschekelendes. Helv Chir Acta 35:556-582
6. Ruedi T, Allgower M (1978) Spätresultate nach operativer Behandlung der Gelenkbrüche am distalen Tibiaende (sog. Pilon- Frakturen). Unfallheilkunde 81: 319-23
7. Maale G, Seligson D (1980) Fractures through the distal weight-bearing surface of the tibia. Orthopedics 3:251-517
8. Mast JW, Spiegel PG, Pappas JN (1988) Fractures of the tibial pilon. Clin Orthop 230:68-82
9. Müller ME, Nazarian S, Koch P, Schatzker J (1990) The comprehensive classification of fractures of long bones. Springer, Berlin Heidelberg New York
10. Crutchfield EH, Seligson D, Henry SL, Warnholtz A (1995) Tibial pilon fractures: a comparative clinical study of management techniques and results. Orthopedics 7:613-17
11. Ruedi TH, Allgower M (1979) Operative treatment of intra-articular fractures of the lower end of the tibia. Clin Orthop 138:105-110
12. Ayeni JP (1988) Pilon fractures of the tibia: a study based on 19 cases. Injury 19:109-114
13. Bourne RB, Rorabeck CH, Macnab BA (1983) Intra-articular fractures of the distal tibia: the pilon fracture. J Trauma 23:591-596
14. Bourne RB (1989) Pilon fractures of the distal tibia. Clin Orthop 240:42-46
15. Mackinnon AP (1928) Fracture of the lower articular surface of the tibia in fracture dislocation of the ankle. J Bone Joint Surg 10:252-262
16. Couvelaire R, Rodier P (1989) Sur une variété de fracture par eclatement du pilon tibial. Rev Orthop 24:329-346
17. Weber BG (1967) Die Verletzung des oberen Sprunggelenkes.1. Auflage. Huber, Bern Stuttgart Wien
18. Weber BG (1972) Die Verletzung des oberen Sprunggelenkes. 2. Auflage. Huber, Bern Stuttgart Wien
19. Heim U (1972) Le traitement chirurgical des fractures du pilon tibial. J Chir 104:307-322
20. Vichard P, Watelet F (1973) Les formes de transition entre les fractures de la malléole interne et les fractures du pilon tibial. Rev Chir Orthop 59:657-665
21. Heim U (1991) Die Pilon Tibial Fraktur. Klassifikation, Operationstechnik, Ergebnisse. Springer, Berlin Heidelberg New York

Imaging of Tibio-Tarsal Joint Injuries

E. Genovese[1], M.G. Angeretti[1], M. Mangini[1], M. Ronga[2], G. Regis[3], C. Fugazzola[1]

The imaging of tibio-tarsal joint injuries varies according to the position and type of injury, which in turn usually depend on the type of accident. Injuries can be divided into either direct or indirect trauma. They both involve, mainly or exclusively, the skeletal apparatus and therefore the most common injuries are fractures. The ligament-capsule structures are frequently also involved particularly in indirect trauma and damage to them may be isolated and responsible for subsequent articular instability [1-4].

Joint imaging is a necessity in this situation, because it is a fundamental tool for accurate diagnosis and for the correct choice of therapeutic strategy [5-8].

Tibio-Tarsal Joint Fractures

A distinction must be made between the different fracture types. Very frequently there are fractures, commonly known as "stress fractures", that are not due to a single accidental event but are to the result of repeated micro-injuries [9, 10].

In order to study and identify a fracture correctly, it is imperative to know the mechanism of injury and the fracture classification. The classification system is somewhat complex, and considers the injury site and how the fracture occurred, the latter being of great importance to the radiologist, and helps identify the type of injury and therefore its location.

A conventional radiological examination is almost always conducted in acute cases where there is pain, swelling and impaired function of the joint. A bone is fractured when there is a break in continuity that characterises a fracture site. Conventional radiology therefore must identify the *basic injury* (Fig.1), and the extent of the fracture line distinguishes between a complete and incomplete injury.

[1]Cattedra di Radiologia, [2]Clinica Ortopedica dell'Università dell'Insubria, Ospedale di Circolo, Fondazione Macchi, Varese; [3]Dipartimento per Immagini ASO CTO, CRF, M. Adelaide, Torino

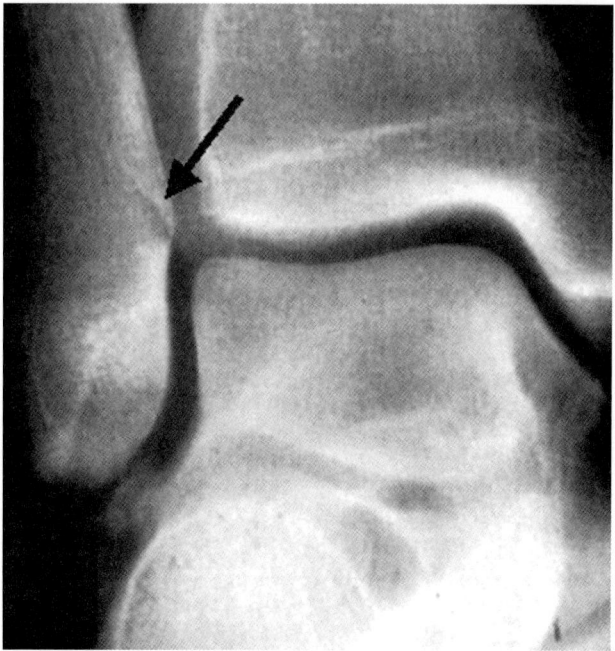

Fig. 1. Conventional antero-posterior X-Ray showing oblique fibular fracture line (*arrow*)

A standard X-Ray allows the various elements of the fracture line to be analysed to establish quickly the degree of severity, and is indispensable for primary treatment. There are various elements of the fracture-line to be considered using conventional radiology.

Basic X-Ray Characteristics

Fracture Extension

Extension of the fracture is one of the first determining factors in the classification between a complete and an incomplete fracture. It identifies a type of injury frequently found in paediatric patients, commonly known as a greenstick fracture. An incomplete fracture is an injury that does not affect the full width of the bone whereas a complete fracture does.

Fracture-Line Direction

Conventional radiology will identify the direction of the fracture-line and differentiate between transverse, oblique, longitudinal and spiral fractures. The choice of therapy can vary according to the direction of the fracture-line, which can also assist in identifying what type of force caused the fracture, e.g. a spiral fracture following rotation of the bone.

Number of Fracture-Lines

A single fracture-line typifies a simple fracture with only two bone fragments. When there are multiple fragments, the fracture is considered complex (Fig. 2) and the number of fragments depends on the number of fracture-lines.

Fracture-Lines and Periskeletal Structures

It is important to examine the relationship that a fracture-line may have with a joint, and identify a fracture that affects the joint or a fracture that affects the capsulo-ligamentous complex. Clearly a fracture-line that affects both is an indication of severity.

When there is more than one fracture-line, it is important to establish the number, appearance, location and quality, to anticipate the likihood of aseptic necrosis due to interruption of the blood supply.

Conventional radiology can identify a necrotic fragment when there have already been changes, such as collapse or sclerosis (Fig. 3). Evaluation of fragment quality is best performed with MRI, which provides excellent definition to determine the status and viability of a fragment (Fig.3).

Computerised tomography (CT) is the best method of examination for fragment morphology. The high degree of resolution demonstrates the smallest fragments (Fig. 4). In some cases it can be difficult to distinguish between an intra- and extra-articular fragment, in which case arthrographic examination by either MRI or CT may be helpful (Fig. 5).

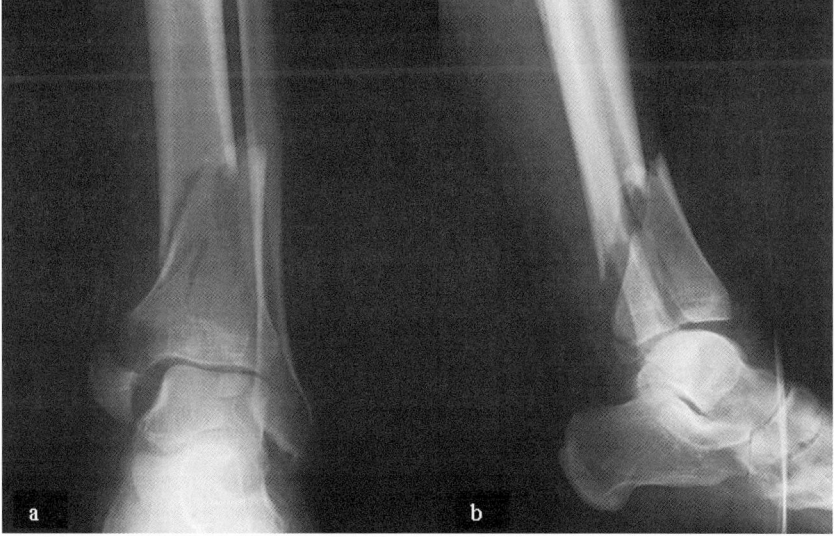

Fig. 2 Conventional X-Rays showing antero-posterior (**a**) and medio-lateral (**b**) views. Complex multi-fragmented fracture affecting the joint

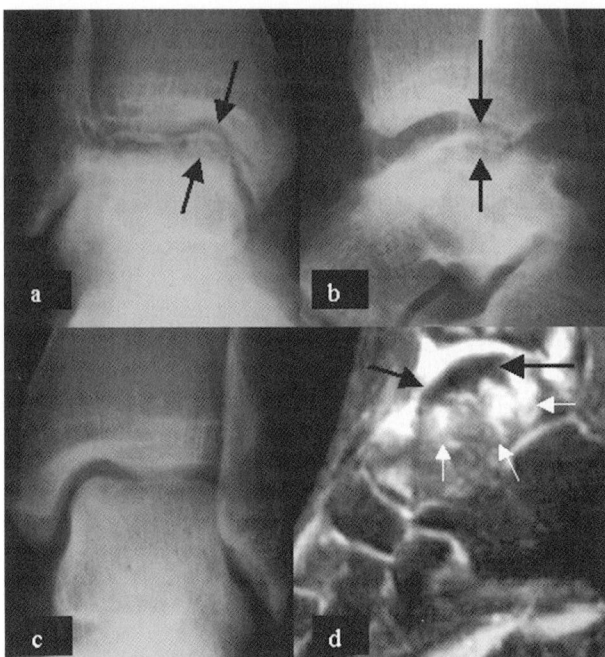

Fig. 3. Conventional antero-posterior X-Rays (a) medio-lateral (b) "collapsed" osteonecrotic sclerotic fragment (*black arrows* in a and b). Conventional X-Ray for comparison of contro-lateral articulation (c). Osteonecrotic fragment seen by MRI (d) as a lifeless image (*black arrows*) which clearly contrasts with the intense reflection of oedema in the cancellous area (*white arrows*)

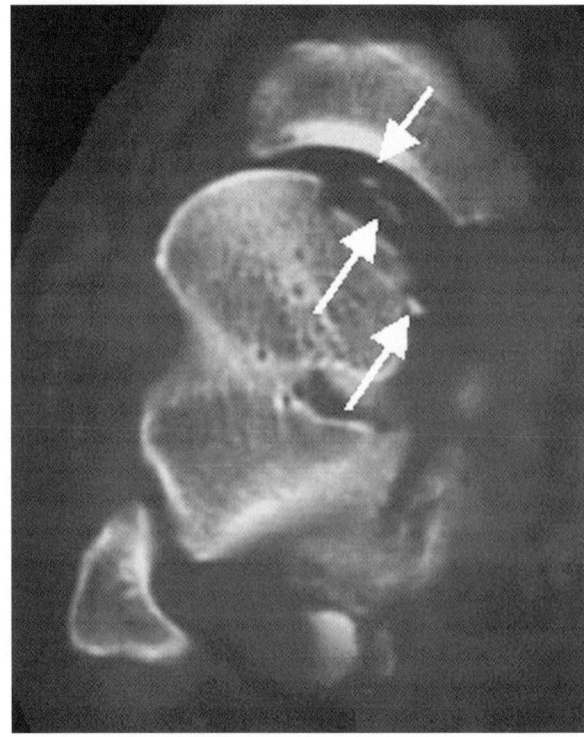

Fig. 4. CT scan showing a fracture of the head of the talus with small fragments (*arrows*)

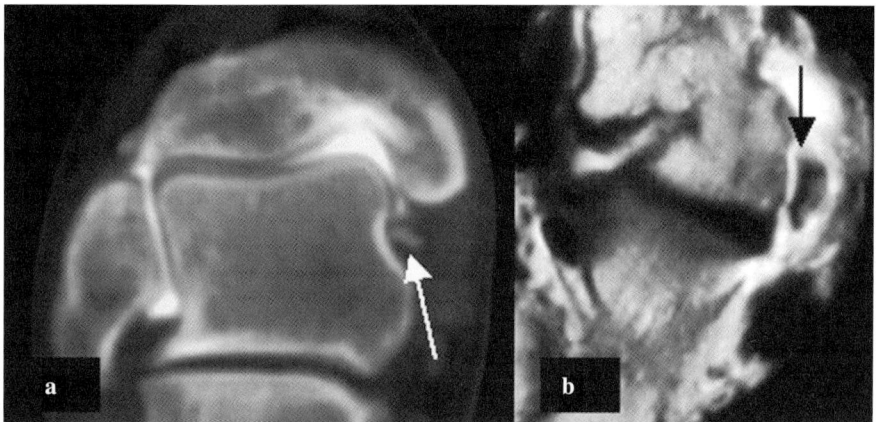

Fig. 5. Arthro-CT (**a**): extra-articular fragment (*white arrow*). Arthro-MR (**b**): intra-articular fragment (*black arrow*)

The tibio-tarsal joint is formed by three bones: the talus, tibia and fibula. Joint stability is provided by ligamentous thickening of the capsule, and there are two systems, lateral and medial, with a further system of four syndesmotic ligaments that maintain tibio-fibular stability. The tibio-tarsal joint is subjected to numerous strains significantly greater than body weight, transmitted by adjacent bones and ligaments. Frequently, indirect loads may damage the ligament-capsule structures or the peri-articular soft tissues [1-3, 11-13].

Fractures

Malleolar Fractures

Three malleoli surround the tibio-tarsal joint: medial, lateral and posterior. The medial and posterior malleoli present respectively the medial and posterior profiles of the distal epiphysis, while the lateral malleolus is formed by the epiphysis of the distal fibula.

There are three different types of malleolar fracture, uni-, bi- and tri-malleolar.

Uni-malleolar fractures can involve the medial or lateral malleoli.

There are other recognised classifications for malleolar fractures but these are the direct consequences of radiological analysis, which demonstrates the importance of imaging for the diagnosis and location of fracture sites, any extensions and the number of different fracture lines that differentiate one injury from another. With conventional radiology using standard views (antero-posterior and lateral) it is possible to identify the elements required to establish a diagnosis and with oblique views, fragment separation and the exact length of fracture-lines.

Tibial Pilon Fractures

These are fractures that affect the distal tibial epiphysis and the articular sur-face. They represent 1% of lower limb fractures and approximately 6% of frac-tures of the tibia. The fibula is involved in 75% of cases [14, 15].

Tibial-pilon fractures are generally a result of high-energy trauma events. Due to the intra-articular damage, the injury has an uncertain prognosis.

There are various classification systems but the role of imaging is estab-lished. Conventional examination can identify and localise an injury, and show fracture-lines and any extension and therefore classify the fracture. There may be multiple fracture lines with comminuted fragments, and the presence of fragments may not be portrayed with any accuracy by conventional radiologi-cal examination, especially if they are very small.

It is the effect of these injuries on joint function that requires a systematic diagnostic approach. Conventional X-Rays cannot establish the number or location of fragments accurately, and CT scanning offers many advantages. Modern computerised tomography equipment allows the patient to be evaluat-ed in one position without having to re-arrange various limbs for a clearer pic-ture, and the new generation of equipment can reconstruct 2D and 3D images. It is this 3-dimensional aspect, which allows an injury to be seen clearly from different angles, that makes this type of imaging indispensable in planning the correct surgical strategy (Fig. 6).

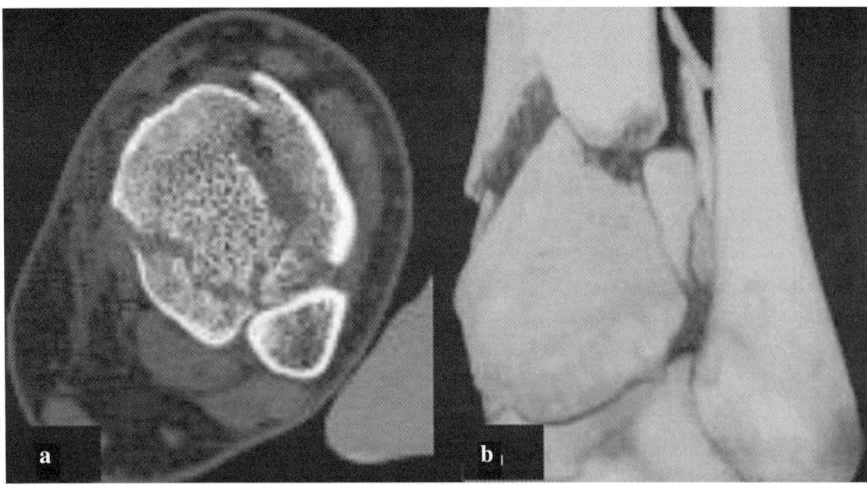

Fig. 6. *Tibial-pilon fractures.* Tomography showing fracture lines (**a**), and 3D reconstruction of the relationship between fracture fragments, showing their displacement (**b**)

MRI is not indicated in "acute" patients, but should be used where the development of osteonecrotic fragments is suspected. The high intrinsic contrast level and especially the difference in "weight" of varied signals with this system, allow it to identify fragment quality accurately. This may help to demonstrate the evolving process of osteonecrosis in a fragment before any of the morphological changes that characterise the later stages. There is debate about the usefulness of MRI in soft tissue lesions (ligament, capsule, muscle, tendon etc.), and when the injury is still recent.

Fractures of the Talus

The mechanism underlying these fractures is dorsi-flexion. When subjected to this type of force, the anterior margin of the tibial pestle impacts with the neck of the talus [9, 16-19].

Because of the pattern of the blood supply to the talus, it is more at risk of osteonecrosis following a fracture of the talar neck, and this will result in clinical complications (Fig. 7). Radiological follow-up of fractures of the talus is important. Classification of fractures of the talar neck highlights the risk of subsequent osteonecrosis (Table 1).

In addition to fractures of the talar neck there can also be fractures of the body (Fig. 8). These are uncommon and frequently associated with malleolar fractures [9, 17]. There are two types, simple (Type I) and comminuted fractures (Type II). The latter is caused by a dorsiflexion injury and tends to involve the lateral process.

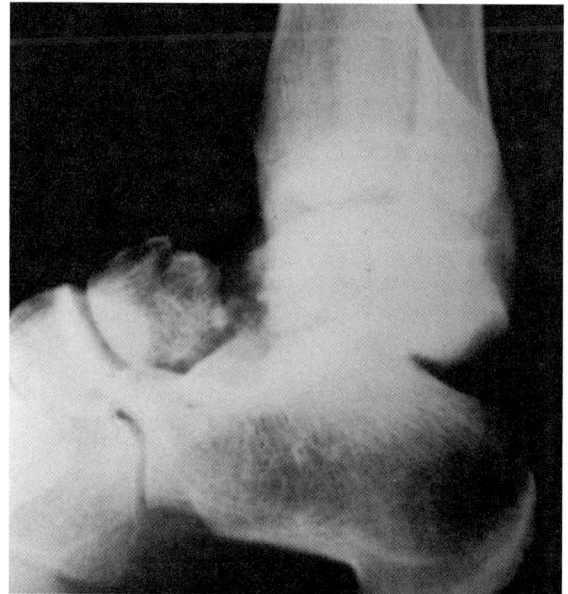

Fig. 7. Fracture of the talar neck

Table 1. Fractures of the talar neck

Type I	Vertical fractures of the neck with involvement of the sub-talar joint without displacement of the body. Osteonecrosis is uncommon
Type II	Vertical fracture of the talar neck with posterior dislocation of the sub-talar joint. There is necrosis in 42% of cases
Type III	Fractures with postero-medial dislocation of the body of the talus from the sub-talar structures. There is necrosis in 90% of cases
Type IV	Is a Type III fracture with, additionally, talo-navicular dislocation. Necrosis may affect the head and the neck

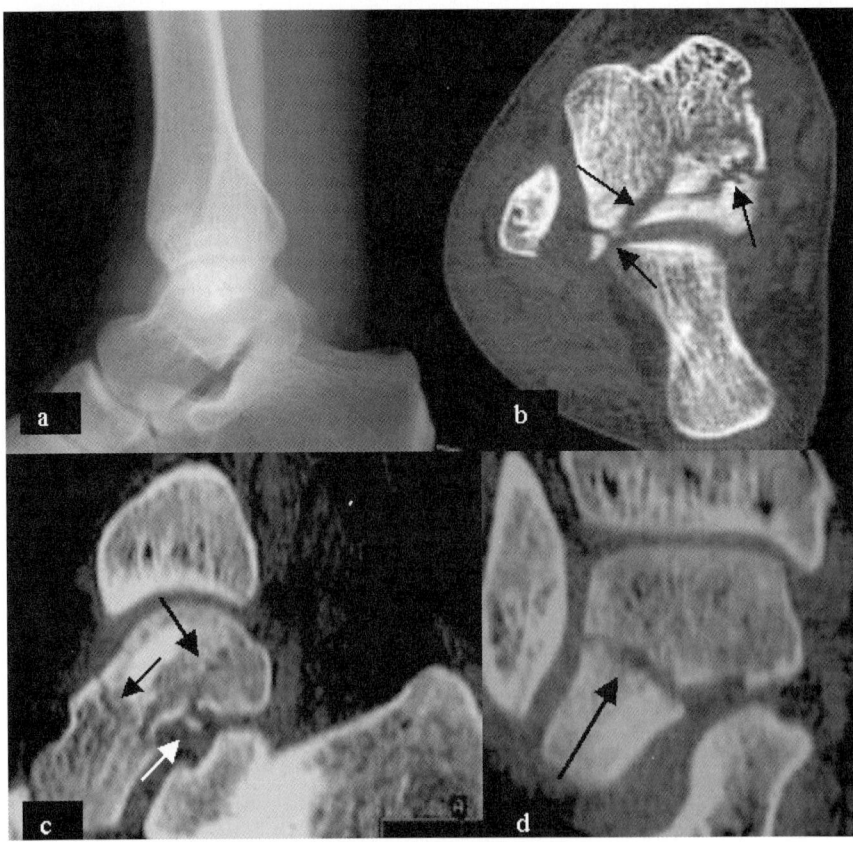

Fig. 8. *Fractures of the talus.* Conventional lateral X-Ray (a) does not demonstrate the fracture lines which are easily identified with CT (*black arrows* in b). 2 dimensional reconstruction (c, d) shows the fracture-line extensions more accurately (*black arrows* in c and d) and the identifies dislocated fragments (*white arrow* in c)

Diagnosis can be achieved by conventional radiology but CT provides a more accurate evaluation of the fracture-pattern.

MRI imaging is preferable for the diagnosis of osteonecrotic complications in the early stages following use of metallic fixation.

Apart from single high energy injuries which fracture the talus, an fatigue fracture of the posterior talar process may occur following repeated micro-trauma. These are "over-use injuries" and are a type of stress fracture [9, 10]. Repetitive flexion-extension movements cause repeated micro-trauma to the posterior talar process with subsequent contusion and oedema of the cancellous bone and an increase in osteoblastic activity resulting in the formation of a fracture-line. In general, these injuries are not detectable by conventional radiography and so are ideal for MRI analysis, which allows assessment of undisplaced injuries. These show up as low intensity images and contrast well in high contrast acquisition with the high intensity signal which characterises bruising and haemorrhagic filling of the bone trabeculae.

Fractures of the Calcaneus

The calcaneus is the most frequently fractured talar bone [19, 20] and is usually the result of a vertical fall, in which it is compressed against the talus which acts as a barrier. It is important to identify these fractures correctly, they are often misinterpreted or underestimated by conventional radiography. Therapeutic strategies and prognoses vary relative to the type of fracture. Classification is according to Böhler's angle, which is obtained by measuring the crossing angle of two lines on a lateral X-Ray image. One from the greater tuberosity and the antero-superior margin, the other from the greater tuberosity to the posterior articular edge. Under normal circumstances, the angle formed by the two lines is between 20° and 40°. In severe fractures, the thalamus is flattened and Böhler's angle is negative. This influences the choice of therapeutic strategy, but immediate surgical intervention is required because of the high risk of osteonecrotic complications.

Table 2. Fractures of calcaneal thalamus

Type I	Fracture into two fragments, undisplaced (antero-internal and postero-external)
Type II	Fracture into two fragments with external displacement of postero-external fragment
Type III	Fractures with three fragments (antero-internal, postero-external and cortico-thalamic)
Type IV	Fractures with four fragments (antero-internal, cortico-thalamic + two postero-external fragments)
Type V	Complex extended fractures

Fractures of the central body require CT investigation to demonstrate the displaced fragments (Fig. 9) and bony collapse that is an important prognostic element, without the need for complicated radiographic projections which are not always easy to carry out in such patients.

The diagnosis of fractures in the other skeletal elements of the tarsus (navicular, cuboid and cuneiform) with standard radiographic techniques is also difficult. Fractures from direct trauma are generally crush injuries, whereas stress or fatigue fractures due to overloading are more frequent and more difficult to identify. MRI is recommended where there are negative radiological results with positive clinical findings (Fig. 10), and can provide very timely information as to the nature of the injury.

With correct sequencing, it is possible to show bruising and haemorrhage in cancellous bone resulting from functional overloading [19, 20].

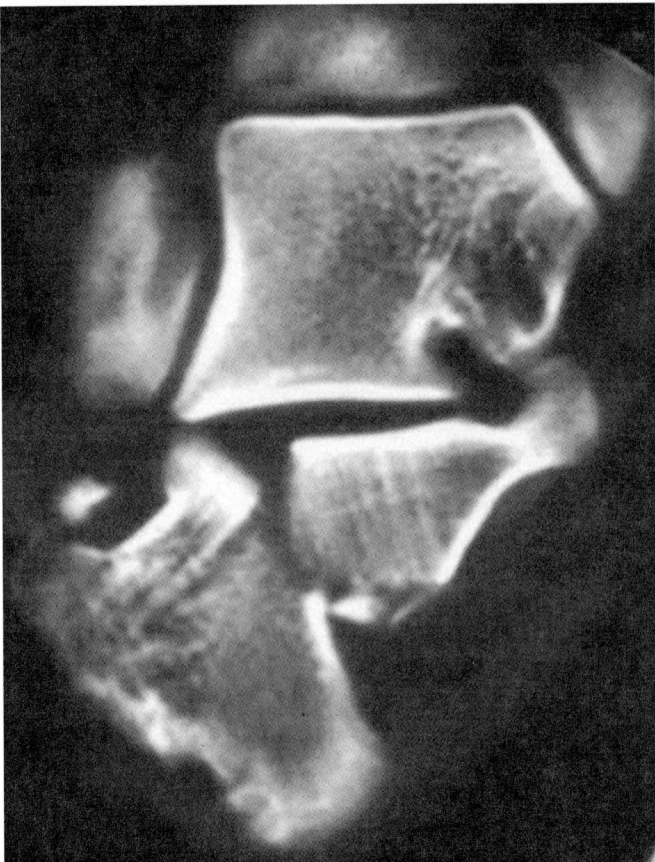

Fig. 9. Fractures of the calcaneus. CT scan showing displaced fracture fragments and collapse of the thalamus

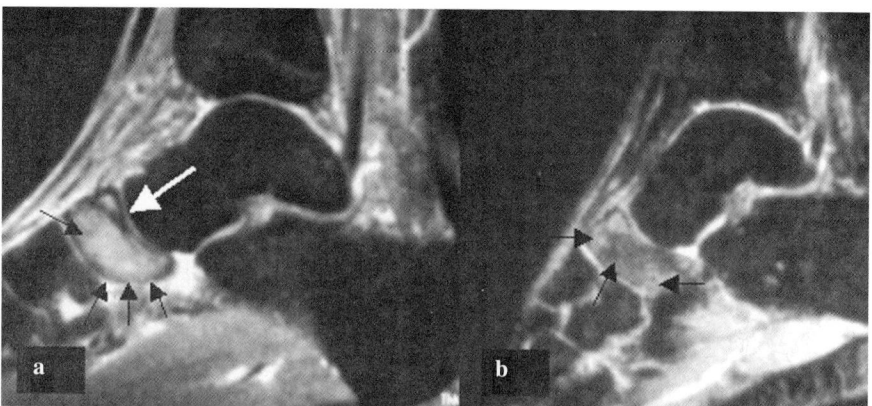

Fig. 10. *Stress fracture of the navicular.* **a** The stress fracture manifests as a low intensity linear image (*white arrow*) under MRI. Bruising and haemorrhagic filling with fat suppression in the cancellous bone gives a high intensity image (*black arrows*). Without enlargement (**b**) the fracture-line cannot be distinguished, but the hyperintensity of the haemorrhage (*black arrows*) indicates the presence of the injury before the the fracture-line becomes visible (stress response)

Ligamento-Capsular Injuries

Trauma through distortion is the most frequent injury to the tibio-tarsal joint (Fig. 11), and mainly involves the external ligament complex that is biomechanically the most exposed.

Injury occurs through forced inversion, whereas eversion-abduction distortion causes injuries to the medial ligaments. Diagnosis is on clinical findings, with peri-malleolar swelling, pain and restricted mobility. It is essential to make an accurate evaluation of the injury and thus establish its exact nature and the presence, if any, of instability in the joint.

Conventional radiology is useful in this type of injury with both standard and dynamic examinations. The standard examination will demonstrate small avulsed fragments.

A dynamic forced inversion examination can demonstrate talar tilt by opening the angle between the upper surface of the talus and the distal tibia. The presence of an angle of tilt greater than 15° is an indirect index of articular instability resulting from injury to the anterior fibulo-talar ligament and the peroneal-calcaneal area of the external collateral ligament (Fig. 12).

Pain and limited mobility are important obstacles in performing a dynamic radiological examination. Ultrasound may be a useful alternative in identifying ligament injuries, as it can show the presence of discontinuity of ligament profiles and identify foreign bodies in joint recesses (Fig. 13). One big advantage of ultrasound is that it can easily be carried out during an inversion load, and demonstrate ligament injury which might not be picked up if the joint is

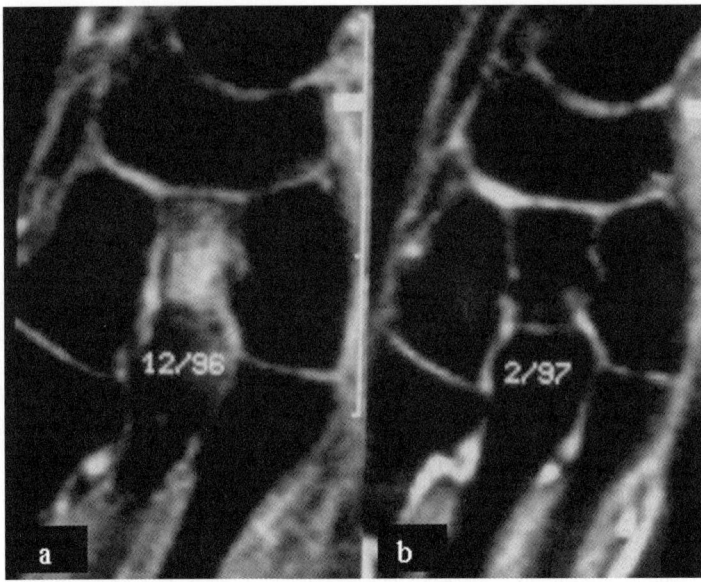

Fig. 11. *Stress fracture of the middle cuneiform.* MRI shows a signal in the images with fat suppression (**a**), bruising in the bony substance but the fracture-line is not distinguishable. A non-enlarged complete view with normal bone signal two months later (**b**)

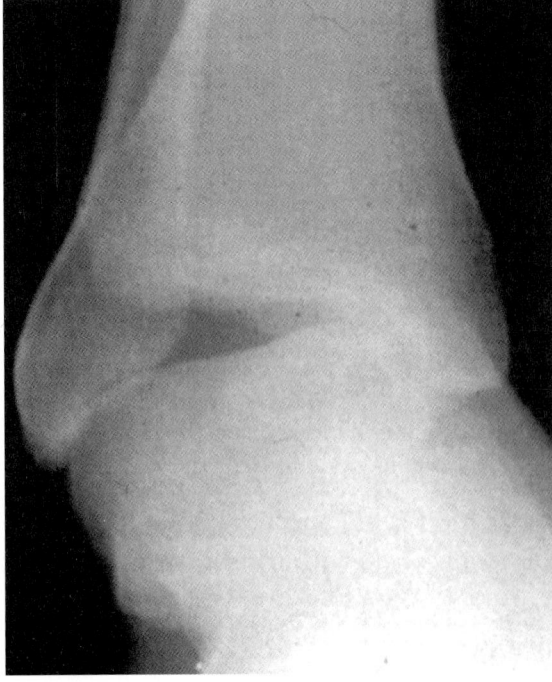

Fig. 12. Antero-posterior view with stress in inversion sho-wing significant talar tilt

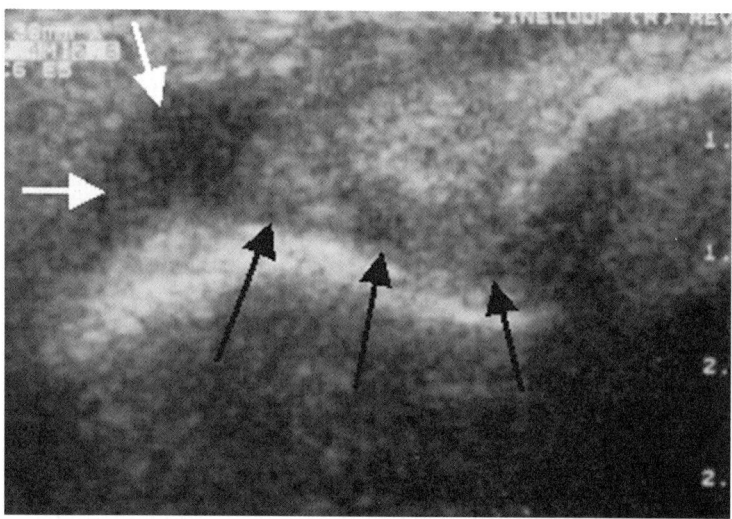

Fig. 13. Ultrasound of the external peri-malleolar region. Lesion the full width of the talar attachment of the anterior peroneo-talar ligament (*black arrows*) with haematoma (*white arrows*)

unloaded. A disadvantage is that it cannot evaluate the underlying bone and osteochondral structures. It is also impossible to identify all the ligament structures along their lengths [21].

A differential diagnosis between partial, distractive and complete lesions is also difficult with CT. The hypointensity governed by depositing and soft tissue bruising masks visualisation of the ligament, at least in the acute phase. The same difficulty in diagnosis occurs with MRI in the subacute phase. Alteration of the signal from haemorrhagic filling at least partially masks visualisation of the ligament tissue, but the widespread focal increase of the signal in T2* acquisition, and the presence of blurred edges is an indirect sign of an incomplete ligament lesion.

An established complete ligament tear is diagnosed by a ligamentous defect, but in the subacute phase is represented by a discontinuation of the ligament in the presence of surrounding haematoma. A safe differential diagnosis between a complete and incomplete ligament lesion is only possible using arthrographic examinations (arthro-CT, arthro-MRI). The contrast medium used in the joint examination is an important diagnostic element and a leakage indicates a complete lesion (Fig. 14). Arthro-CT or arthro-MRI can also accurately establish the intra-articular position of a fragment that behaves like an "island" surrounded by contrast medium [2-4, 13, 22, 23].

A regular consequence of one or more sprain injuries is articular instability and this produces progressive wear and tear on the cartilage profile, particularly the talar dome and adjacent tibial articular surface. Articular instability

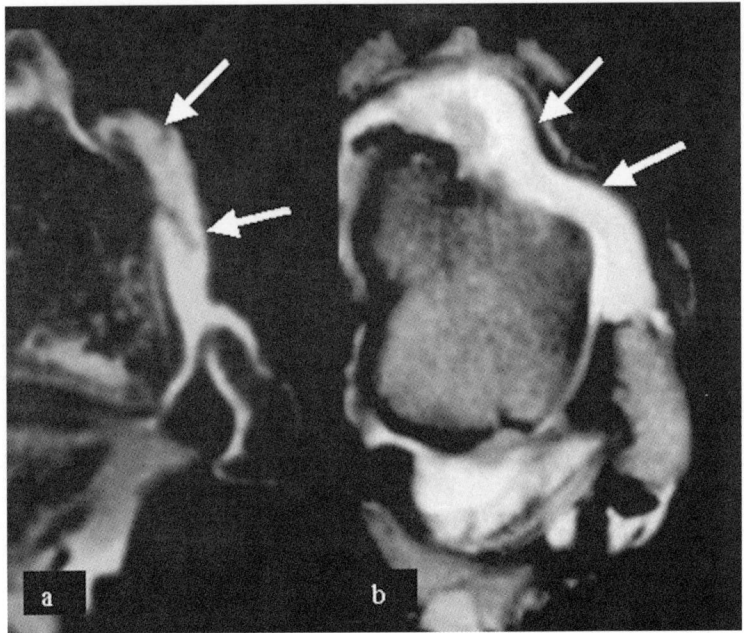

Fig. 14. Complete lesion of the anterior talo-fibular ligament by arthro-CT (**a**) and arthro-MRI (**b**). Contrast medium leakage to extra-articular site is indicated (*arrows*)

with the resultant impaired loading can lead to the onset of osteochondral lesions [24-26], the identification of which is straight forward with conventional radiology but it is not satisfactory for fragment quality or stability. It is therefore not possible to grade the injury correctly.

Osteochondral fragment quality can be studied satisfactorily using MRI. The signal analysis will differentiate a fragment with a skeletal-type signal intensity or a fragment with haemorrhagic or just hypovascular fibrous contents.

Peri-lesional bone damage can be demonstrated clearly with MRI but only an arthrographic examination will show the difference between a stable and unstable fragment (Fig. 15).

The passage of contrast medium along the continuity of the cartilaginous profile, and the comparison between fragment and healthy bone readings indicate the degree of fragment instability.

In conclusion, in cases of acute trauma of the tibio-tarsal joint, conventional radiology with suitable framing is sufficient to identify fracture sites and types. CT however is preferable in traumatised patients for its clear advantages, particularly the possibility of reconstructing 2D and 3D images which are indispensable for accurate therapeutic planning to guide surgical osteosynthesis.

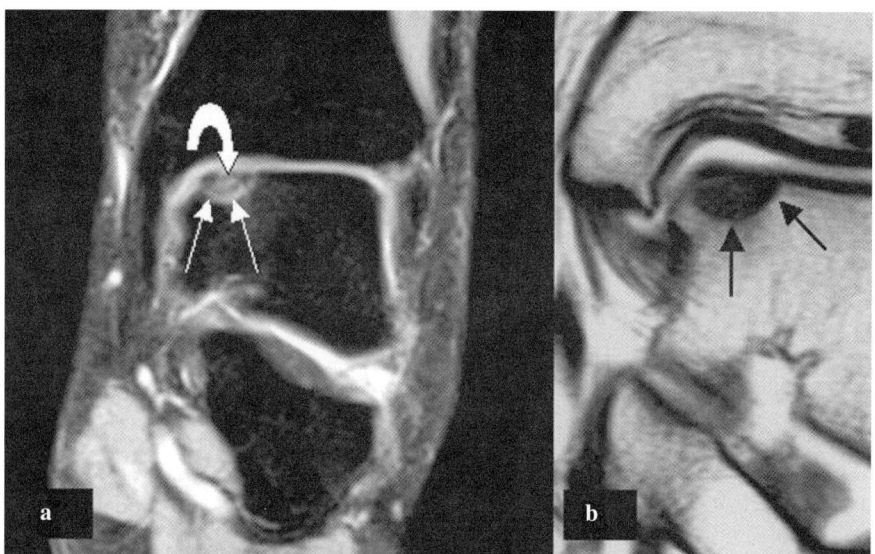

Fig. 15. Osteochondral lesion of the talar dome. MR imaging clearly shows the intense signal of the fragment surrounded by haemorrhagic content (*curved arrow in a*). The fragment is clearly encapsulated by lines (*white arrow in a*); a granular wall can be seen where the two surfaces meet. In arthrographic MRI, the hyper-intense contrast medium used does not infiltrate between fragments and healthy bone (*black arrow in b*) and therefore, the lesion is stable. In distorted lesions, imaging plays a somewhat limited role, but is of great help in identifying elementary lesions that are the basis of chronic post-traumatic instability

The role of MRI is limited to fracture follow-up with the aim of early iden-tification of any osteonecrotic complications. On the other hand, the role of MRI is of the highest importance in acute injuries not visible to conventional radiology, bone contusion and lesions caused by repeated micro-trauma and stress fractures.

In distorsive lesions, imaging plays a somewhat limited role, but is of great help in identifying elementary lesions that are the basis of chronic post-traumatic instability.

References

1. Zimmer TJ (1991) Chronic and recurrent ankle sprains. Clin Sports Med 10(3):653-659
2. Cheung Y, Rosenberg ZS (2001) MR imaging of ligamentous abnormalities of the ankle and foot. Magn Reson Imaging Clin N Am 9(3):507-531
3. Cardone BW, Erickson SJ, Den Hartog BD, Carrera GF (1993) MRI of injury to the lateral collateral ligamentous complex of the ankle. J Comput Assist Tomogr 17(1):102-107
4. Erickson SJ, Smith JW, Ruiz ME et al (1991) MR imaging of the lateral collateral liga-ment of the ankle. Am J Roentgenol 156(1):131-136

5. Zanetti M, De Simoni C, Wetz HH et al (1997) Magnetic resonance imaging of injuries to the ankle joint: can it predict clinical outcome? Skeletal Radiol 26(2):82-88
6. Daffner RH (1994) Ankle trauma. Semin Roentgenol 29(2):134-151
7. Lazarus ML (1999) Imaging of the foot and ankle in the injured athlete. Med Sci Sports Exerc 31[Suppl 7]:412-420
8. Bencardino J, Rosenberg ZS, Delfaut E (1999) MR imaging in sports injuries of the foot and ankle. Magn Reson Imaging Clin N Am 7(1):131-149
9. Bradshaw C, Khan K, Brukner P (1996) Stress fracture of the body of the talus in athletes demonstrated with computer tomography. Clin J Sport Med 6(1):48-51
10. Spitz DJ, Newberg AH (2002) Imaging of stress fractures in the athlete. Radiol Clin North Am 40(2):313-331
11. Lubin JW, Miller RA, Robinson BJ, Blevins FT (2000) Achilles tendon rupture associated with ankle fracture. Am J Orthop 29(9):707-708
12. Stevens MA, El-Khoury GY, Kathol MH et al (1999) Imaging features of avulsion injuries. Radiographics 19(3):655-672
13. Tochigi Y, Yoshinaga K, Wada Y, Moriya H (1998) Acute inversion injury of the ankle: magnetic resonance imaging and clinical outcomes. Foot Ankle Int 19(11):730-734
14. Robinson P, Whitehouse RW, Freemont AJ, Ellis D (2001) Synovial osteochondromatosis complicating pilon fracture of the tibia. Skeletal Radiol 30(8):475-477
15. Mainwaring BL, Daffner RH, Riemer BL (1988) Pilon fractures of the ankle: a distinct clinical and radiologic entity. Radiology 168(1):215-218
16. Anderson IF, Crichton KJ, Grattan-Smith T et al (1989) Osteochondral fractures of the dome of the talus. J Bone Joint Surg Am 71(8):1143-1152
17. Thordarson DB (2001) Talar body fractures. Orthop Clin North Am 32(1):65-77
18. Wechsler RJ, Schweitzer ME, Karasick D et al (1997) Helical CT of talar fractures. Skeletal Radiol 26(3):137-142
19. Hindman BW, Ross SD, Sowerby MR (1986) Fractures of the talus and calcaneus: evaluation by computed tomography. J Comput Tomogr 10(2):191-196
20. Zeiss J, Ebraheim N, Rusin J, Coombs RJ (1991) Magnetic resonance imaging of the calcaneus: normal anatomy and application in calcaneal fractures. Foot Ankle 11(5):264-273
21. Morvan G, Busson J, Wybier M, Mathieu P (2001) Ultrasound of the ankle. Eur J Ultrasound 14(1):73-82
22. Faletti C, De Stefano N, Regis G et al (1995) Magnetic resonance arthrography. Preliminary experience in study technic and main diagnostic applications. Radiol Med 89(3):211-214
23. Cheung Y, Rosenberg ZS, Magee T, Chinitz L (1992) Normal anatomy and pathologic conditions of ankle tendons: current imaging techniques. Radiographics 12(3):429-444
24. Loredo R, Sanders TG (2001) Imaging of osteochondral injuries. Clin Sports Med 20(2):249-278
25. Sijbrandij ES, van Gils AP, Louwerens JW, de Lange EE (2000) Post-traumatic subchondral bone contusions and fractures of the talotibial joint: occurrence of "kissing" lesions. Am J Roentgenol 175(6):1707-1710
26. Labovitz JM, Schweitzer ME (1998) Occult osseous injuries after ankle sprains: incidence, location, pattern, and age. Foot Ankle Int 19(10):661-667

Closed Fractures

Type V. Crushing injury to the physis generally in isolation or associated with a Type II displacement, occasionally with Types III or IV or in severe cases of polytrauma. It does not have characteristics that allow for diagnosis acutely nor can it be suspected just on the basis of a trauma (violent contusions, falls etc.).

Injury Mechanisms

As in adult malleolar fractures, there are various classification systems for tibio-tarsal epiphyseal injuries based on the mechanisms leading to the injury. The widely-used in clinical practice is Crenshaw's classification [6-10] that describes five different types of fracture mechanism. The important thing about a classification system of this kind is that it influences the type of treatment to be administered, particularly reduction.

1. *Abduction.* This mechanism is frequently responsible for injuries, mostly Type II displacements, where the epiphysis is laterally displaced with lateral or posterior metaphyseal fragmentation. They are associated with fibular metaphyseal or diaphyseal fractures. Reduction is simple, prognosis is good as only shear forces come into play with no compression of the physis.

2. *External rotation.* Forced external rotation of the foot is the most frequent cause of a Type II displacement with metaphyseal fragmentation and posterior, sometimes substantial displacement of the epiphysis. It is usually associated with a diaphyseal fracture of the fibula, and the prognosis is generally good. It is the same mechanism that causes Type IV injuries (triplanar fractures) in which the epiphyseal or epiphyseal-metaphyseal fragment stays mostly attached to the fibula. In adolescent patients nearing closure of the physis, external rotation can result in a juvenile Tillaux fracture with lateral epiphyseal fragments, that usually remain connected to the fibula.

3. *Plantar flexion.* This can produce a Type II tibial injury with posterior metaphyseal fragmentation, posterior epiphyseal displacement, and an intact fibula. The prognosis is good.

4. *Axial compression and direct trauma.* These are high energy injuries (rolling, falls etc.) with frequent associated polytrauma. Damage to the physis can pass unnoticed but often has a Type V component. Prognosis is poor.

5. *Adduction.* Types III and IV medial injuries are caused by this mechanism. The fracture is caused by direct compression of the tibial malleolus by part of the body of the talus, which with progressive abduction involves the physeal cartilage with possible Type V damage. Prognosis may be poor even after precise reduction. However, displacement is always apparent and is associated with displacement of the fibular malleolus.

6. *Internal rotation* is an unusual mechanism responsible for a rarely seen form of tri-planar fracture which would be a Type IV injury.

Clinical Diagnosis

The tibio-tarsal region is not frequently involved in bony injury in early child-hood (1.6% of all the Authors' case histories) [11]. They are almost always "green stick" or "buckling" supramalleolar injuries. It is only from 8 years that this region becomes more frequently involved but, however, it only represents 3.4% of all fractures in the paediatric age group. Boys more commonly suffer these injuries [11].

Diagnosis is based on a history of recent trauma, physical examination and X-Rays. The examination may show a very obvious deformity while at other times there may only be a small swelling with specific sites of pain, suggesting an undisplaced epiphyseal injury of the tibia or fibula. Nowadays, traditional radiology is frequently supplemented by CT examination for precise diagnosis of complex fractures (tri-plane fractures) [12, 13].

Treatment

The treatment of tibio-tarsal fractures at paediatric age should be aimed mostly at repairing tibial damage and secondly at tibio-fibular syndesmosis. Reduction of a fibular injury and restoration of fibular length would seem to be less impor-tant than in adult trauma treatment. There are no reports in the literature about negative outcomes to early epiphysiodesis with shortening or axial deviation of the fibula, nor of persistent tibio-tarsal instability due to impairment of the tibio-fibular ligaments. It is probably for this reason that for most tibio-tarsal injuries conservative orthopaedic treatment is sufficient. The treatment of single epiphyseal tibial displacements will now be considered.

Types I and II. Surgical reduction is carried out under sedation or general anaesthetic according to the patient's condition [14]. The aim is to return the epiphyseal fragment to its natural site. It is for this reason, as mentioned ear-lier, that it is important to understand the mechanism of injury. Orthopaedic treatment is always possible, and frequently the most marked displacements can be reduced with light traction. This is associated with injury mechanisms such as abduction, extension or internal rotation of the foot. In exceptional cases of Type II injury, displacement of the periosteum or soft tissue makes surgerical intervention necessary [15]. Even incomplete reduction may be suf-ficient for an residual angular deformity up to 15° of valgus and procurvatum. The same applies for translation deformities, even if more than 25% of the thickness of the diaphysis, considering the age of the patient and the poten-tial for subsequent growth and correction (this being somewhat modest after 12-13 years of age) [12]. Angular deformity of the distal tibial of this type (unlike the proximal tibia) is not clinically very evident and is quickly cor-rected in the months following the accident. To avoid residual varus deformi-ty, which is not well tolerated and tends less towards spontaneous correction, reduction is maintained with a full length groin-to-toe plaster cast for 30 days non weightbearing, with the foot, if necessary, slightly raised. Clinically relevant shortening or lengthening (more than 1 cm) are somewhat rare events.

Types III and IV. Physeal and articular surface damage are associated injuries. Orthopaedic treatment is required in displaced fractures. Because of possible unsatisfactory outcomes, particular attention should be paid to epiphyseal displacement of the tibial malleolus. Definite differential diagnosis between Types III and IV is not always possible (as seen even in McFarland's original sketches) as the metaphyseal fragment is often very small and not visible by radiology. These injuries must be perfectly reduced. The definition of 2 mm as the maximum allowable diastasis would not seem applicable, as the fracture plane is frequently not perfectly orthogonal for X-Ray purposes and because there is almost always associated malleolar rotation in the frontal plane with partial over-positioning of the fractured bone [16, 17]. It has been demonstrated that a fracture line with diastasis at the physeal level in any bone is filled with newly-formed bone tissue, producing therefore an area of epiphysiodesis.

Orthopaedic treatment is therefore only indicated for completely displaced fractures while reduction and surgical synthesis are obligatory for the other types. The operation is carried out by a short medial anterior incision with the joint being opened at the level of the fracture site to inspect completed reduction. Debridement of the fracture site and malleolar periosteal stripping are not advisable because of the danger of damage to the physis and osteogenic perichondrium. Synthesis is carried out using two K-wires or in the author's preference, with a horizontally positioned cannulated epiphyseal screw and washer [17, 18]. A screw or cross-fixing K-wire should only be used when necessary (e.g. when there is a small medial fragment). The limb is then put in plaster cast and maintained without weightbearing for 30 days. The screw can be removed after another 30-60 days.

Fractures of the lateral epiphysis, that is juvenile Tillaux and tri-plane fractures, have a better prognosis, as the patient population is of a higher average age with fewer potential consequences to changes in growth. Surgical reduction can be attempted with caution in these patients to obtain good articular surface reconstruction and a CT scan check should be carried out after the reduction, if possible. A possible diastasis at articular cartilage level may cause the rare complication of defective intra-articular callus formation. Surgical reduction and synthesis with screws (always parallel to the physeal line) could also be indicated in these cases [17].

Outcomes

Two features of epiphyseal displacement of the ankle will influence the outcome of these injuries: physeal growth cartilage is involved, and this will have an effect on future distal tibial and fibular growth; a disturbance of continuity is created in fracture Types III and IV in both the physeal and articular cartilage. Possible consequences over time will be changes in the growth pattern with shortening and/or angular deviation and articular irregularities with the risk of post-traumatic arthrosis [19].

The distal tibial growth plate provides for 40-45% of the overall growth of this segment; the tibial physis can develop post-traumatic growth disturbance which is less common in the fibular physis (probably due to the benign nature of Type I and II injuries). This discrepancy can lead to changes in the relationship in the distal tibia and fibula, where radiographically, the fibular physis is situated at the level of the articular tibio-talar joint line.

Alteration in tibial growth is almost always a consequence of Type IV epiphyseal displacement (McFarland's fracture); it is rare in Type III and even less common but possible in Type II. Two causes are recognised: inadequate reduction of an epiphyseal fracture with the consequent formation of a epiphysiodesis bone bridge, or the presence of a Type V element which is almost always diagnosed later [14]. An injury of this type must always be suspected in cases of violent trauma or polytrauma or when associated with fractures of the body of the talus or crushing fractures of the distal tibial epiphysis. However, Type V displacement in juvenile Tillaux or tri-plane fractures is rare, and is due to a rotational mechanism with shearing forces on the physeal cartilage. Other concomitant causes for post-traumatic epiphysiodesis are surgery to the fracture site, transfixation osteosynthesis and possible septic complications.

If epiphysiodesis is carried out on the physis, it will cause shortening of the tibia. If it occurs round the margins of the gworth plate, it will cause axial tibiotarsal deviation, almost always varus to which an element of shortening will be superimposed. Isolated shortening of the tibia will lead to relative fibular lengthening with progressive distal displacement of the malleolus and subsequent varus deviation of the foot [20].

Irregular healing of the joint surface, which can happen in, medial and lateral Types III and IV epiphyseal injuries, is rare but important, because of possible development of post-traumatic arthrosis. Evaluating the potential sequelae of these injuries is difficult, with consideration of an early operation to improve the articular surface and whether or not to perform an epiphysiodesis.

In conclusion, even the best reduction or the most stable synthesis is no guarantee of complication-free treatment. The patients' parents must always be informed about possible complications and regular follow-up is mandatory (six-monthly or yearly) to check on growth for at least two years, and changes in epiphyseal function have been recorded 4 years after injury [16].

Treatment of Outcomes

The primary treatment of post-traumatic epiphysiodesis of the ankle is to remove the bony bridge and replace it with biologically inert material (adipose tissue, silastic, polymethylmethacrylate) [21, 22]. Indications for this treatment possible are an area of epiphysiodesis which is visible on X-Ray and occupies no more than 50% of the growth plate in a patient with at least one year of residual growth remaining.

The bone bridge must be precisely defined, and can be removed in a minimally invasive manner by excavating it with a drill and then replacing it with inert material using the same access point. Another choice would be to carry out a distraction procedure using a fine wire fixator to produce epiphyseal separation. At this point, a small incision allows the area of the epiphysiodesis to be explored and cleared and the gap filled with adipose tissue.

Although this is a logical treatment, reported results are variable and sometimes disappointing. Spontaneous breaking of the bone bridge has been reported in younger children with subsequent limited growth, but this is not a foreseeable phenomenon and is not to be counted on [14].

Angular correction is indicated to prevent the onset of post-traumatic tibiotarsal arthrosis. The more usual varus deformity is treated by early medial tibial supramalleolar osteotomy. Minimal fixation with staples or K-wires and a plastercast (Fig. 2) is usually sufficient. If the injury is not severe, this operation

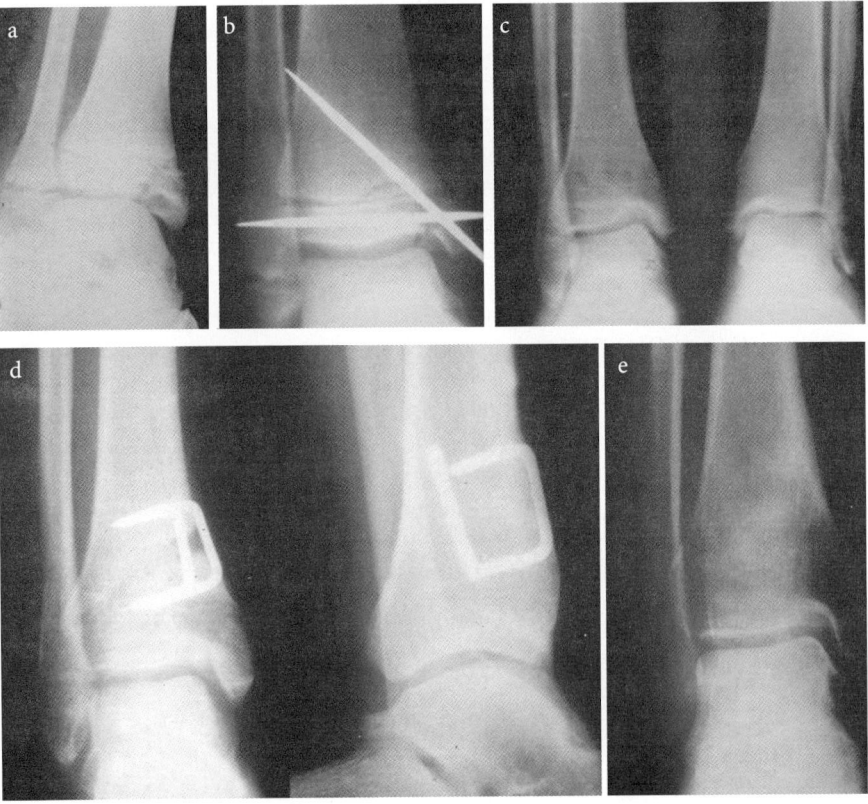

Fig. 2. a Type III epiphyseal displacement. **b** Percutaneous synthesis using K-wires. **c** At the age of 14 tibio-tarsal varus deviation after post-traumatic medial epiphysiodesis. **d** Growth cartilage obliterated. Supramalleolar wedge osteotomy followed by minimal synthesis with staples and plastercast. **e** A follow-up visit after 12 years shows no signs of arthrosis. Patient asymptomatic

is better carried out towards the end of the growth period, thus avoiding relapse of the asymmetrical growth.

When there is isolated tibial shortening of 3 cm or axial deviation associated with shortening, correction with or without lengthening with external fixation is indicated [14, 19]. Axial malalignment can be complex and in an oblique plane. This would suggest employing the Ilizarov method, because the fine wire fixation takes up a minimum of space and the fixation allows for micrometric angular correction during or after lengthening. Using this method, the normal relationship of the tibio-fibular pestle can be restored when there is relative fibular lengthening. The final length discrepancy will not be more than 10 cm, so one operation towards the end of the growth period is sufficient and also ensures better collaboration from an adolescent patient who is well motivated and willing to cooperate. Possible complications are well described: infections from the method of fixation, knee stiffness and foot equinus occur in proportion to the degree of discrepancy to be corrected.

References

1. Dias LS, Giegerich CR (1983) Fractures of the distal tibial epiphysis in adolescence. J Bone Joint Surg Am 65:438-444
2. Köhler A, Zimmer EA (1970) Limiti del normale ed inizio del patologico nella diagnostica radiologica dello scheletro. Ambrosiana, Milano
3. Mac Nealy GA, Rogers LF, Hernandez R, Poznanski AK (1982) Injuries of the distal tibial epiphysis: systematic radiographic evaluation. Am J Roentgenol 138(4):683-689
4. Ogden JA, Lee J (1990) Accessory ossification patterns and injuries of the malleoli. J Pediatr Orthop 10:306-316
5. Salter RB, Harris R (1963) Injuries involving the epiphyseal plate. J Bone Joint Surg Am 45:587-622
6. Onimus M (1990) Les fractures de la cheville. In: Clavert JM, Metaizeau JP (eds) Les fractures des membres chez l'enfant. Sauramps, Montpellier, pp 357-368
7. Marmor L (1970) An unusual fracture of the tibial epiphysis. Clin Orthop 73:132-135
8. Von Laer L (1985) Classification, diagnosis and treatment of transitional fractures of the distal part of the tibia. J Bone Joint Surg Am 67:687-698
9. Khouri N, Ducloyer Ph, Carlioz H (1989) Fractures triplane de la cheville. Rev Chir Orthop 75:394-404
10. Crenshaw AH (1965) Injuries of the distal tibial epiphysis. Clin Orthop 41:98-107
11. Mastragostino S, Carbone M, Origo C (1991) La traumatologia degli arti e della colonna vertebrale in età pediatrica. In: Tamisani AM, Magillo P (eds) Gli infortuni in età pediatrica. Proceedings of the 1st Meeting "La traumatologia degli arti e della colonna celebrale", Genova, pp 34-46
12. Rockwood CA, Wilkins KE, King RE (1991) Fractures in children, Vol 3. Lippincott, Philadelphia
13. Leitch JM, Cundy PJ, Paterson DC (1989) Three-dimensional imaging of a juvenile Tillaux fracture. J Pediatr Orthop 9:602-603
14. Mastragostino S, Stella G, Scarsi M et al (1992) Lesioni ossee traumatiche della tibiotarsica in età evolutiva. Minerva Ortop Traumatol 43:183-188

15. Grace DL (1983) Irreducible fracture-separations of the distal tibial epiphysis. J Bone Joint Surg Br 65:160-162
16. Kling TF, Bright RW, Hensinger RN (1984) Distal tibial physeal fractures in children that may require open reduction. J Bone Joint Surg Am 66:647-657
17. Kling TF (1990) Operative treatment of ankle fractures in children. Orthop Clin North Am 21:381-392
18. Carbone M, Boero S, Scarsi M, Stella G (1992) Le lesioni ossee traumatiche della tibiotarsica in età pediatrica. Chirurgia del piede 16:355-358
19. Filipe G (1990) Sequelles des fractures du cou-de-pied de l'enfant. In: Clavert JM, Metaizeau JP (eds) Les fractures des membres chez l'enfant. Sauramps, Montpellier, pp 369-376
20. Kärrholm J, Hansson LI, Selvik G (1984) Changes in tibiofibular relationships due to growth disturbances after ankle fractures in children. J Bone Joint Surg Am 66:1198-1210
21. Bright RW (1974) Operative correction of partial epiphyseal plate closure by osseous-bridge resection and silicone-rubber implant. J Bone Joint Surg Am 56:655-664
22. Langenskiöld A (1975) An operation for partial closure of an epiphyseal plate in children, and its experimental basis. J Bone Joint Surg Br 57:325-330

Treatment Criteria for Closed Injuries

L. Renzi Brivio, A.L. Pizzoli

Introduction

The term tibial pilon was first used by the French radiologist Destot in 1911 to identify the anatomical region corresponding to the distal third of the tibia, extending proximally approximately 5 cm from the joint line. The term tibial pilon fracture (7-10% of tibial fractures) is used to define a group of injuries that always involves the distal tibial articular surface with, in 85% of cases, fractures of the fibula, and should be distinguished from malleolar injuries which also involve the metaphyseal region [1, 2]. Tibial-pilon fractures may be caused by low-energy rotational injuries such as sports accidents or can be high-energy complex trauma, frequently caused by road traffic accidents or falls from a height. The injuries may present with comminution and articular or metaphyseal displacement to a greater or lesser extent, with possible diaphyseal extension and/or severe soft tissue damage, and may or may not be open. For this reason, careful history and pre-operative examination is indispensable for choosing the correct therapeutic strategy.

As with all articular fractures, anatomical reduction and stabilisation of the fracture site is required through the entire healing process period to guarantee a good long-term result. These objectives are not always easy to achieve considering the quality of the local bone tissue, which is mainly cancellous and frequently osteopoenic. The surgeon's first task therefore is that of gathering all the clinical and instrumental data available regarding the injury, in order to choose the most effective surgical option, especially in terms of limiting possible local complications (fragment osteonecrosis, fracture site infection, delayed union, post-surgical soft tissue damage, joint stiffness) [1-3].

Divisione di Ortopedia e Traumatologia, Ospedale C. Poma, Mantova

Decision Criteria

There are four main criteria regarding choice of treatment for tibial-pilon fractures:
-   qualitative and quantitative evaluation of the trauma event (high or low-energy);
-   morphological evaluation of the osseous and/or osteochondral injury;
-   evaluation of the effects on peripheral soft tissue;
-   presence of concomitant illnesses (diabetes, vascular disease etc.).

The first point is extremely important as it influences the vitality of bone fragments and soft tissue even distant from the fracture site. It is also considered when choosing the surgical approach and type of fixation to be employed. With high-energy injuries the local vascular circulation is frequently compromised as a direct result of the injury, and local haematoma, oedema and fracture blisters require the least invasive surgical approach possible, relative to the morphology of the fracture. Diagnosis and prognosis are based on standard radiographic and CT scans (with possible 2D and 3D reconstruction). The Ruedi and Allgower classification is certainly the simplest and most widely used system to this end (Fig. 1):
-   Type I fractures are generally secondary to low-energy trauma events, involving the joint line but without fragment displacement;
-   Type II fractures involve the joint and there is fragment displacement but no articular or metaphyseal comminution;
-   Type III fractures involve both comminution and displacement with a loss of cancellous bone substance in the metaphyseal region.

The AO classification system (Fig. 2) similarly differentiates the varying injuries morphologically into sub-groups 43-B (partial articular fractures) and 43-C (complete articular fractures) where B1 and C1 correspond approximately to the Ruedi and Allgower Type I, B2 and C2 to Type II, and B3 and C3 to Type III [3-5]. Both classification systems quantify the prognosis by determining the degrees of comminution and articular involvement. When choosing a treatment regime, there are essentially two types of injury to be considered: *simple fractures* which include Ruedi and Allgower Types I and II, and *complex fractures* which include Type III.

The condition of the soft tissues should be carefully evaluated, as the patient's condition will change over time, and the appearance of the skin does not always correspond to the situation subcutaneously. The most widely-used classification system for this type of assessment is that proposed by Tscherne:
-   Grades 0 and I injuries are secondary to low-energy trauma and are characterised by absent or surface changes in the skin without disturbance of continuity;
-   Grade II injuries are secondary to high-energy trauma with deep, contaminated abrasions, blisters, significant bruising and a clinical picture suggesting impending compartment syndrome;

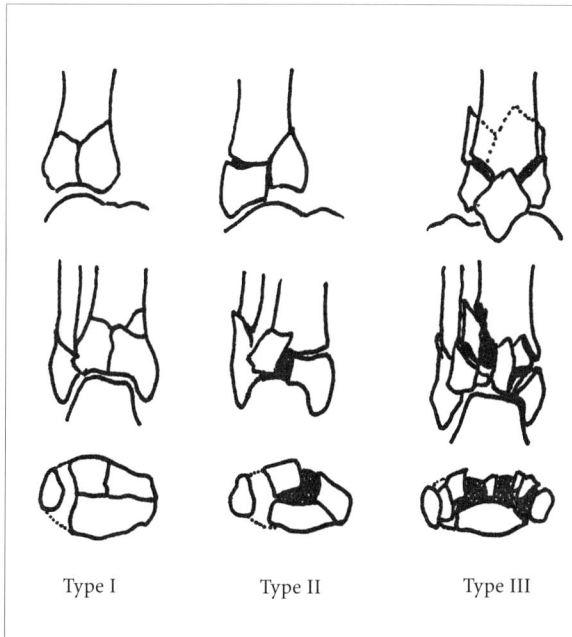

Fig. 1. The Ruedi-Allgower tibial-pilon fracture classification. *Type I:* articular fracture (undisplaced). *Type II:* articular fracture, displacement but no comminution. *Type III:* articular fracture displacement and comminution

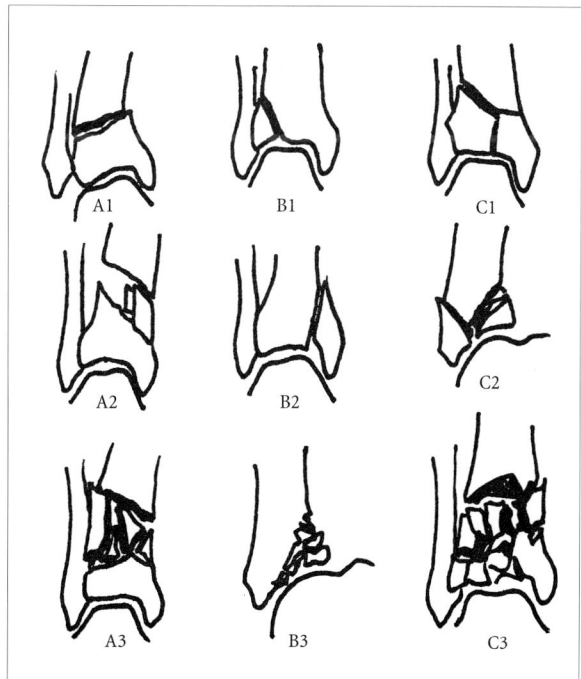

Fig. 2. The AO/ASIF distal-tibial fracture classification. *Type 43-A:* extra-articular fracture. *Type 43-B:* fractures involving an articular sector. *Type 43-C:* fractures globally involving the joint

- Grade III injuries are secondary to contusion or direct crushing. These injuries are associated with Type II skin damage, ischaemic muscle damage and the presence of possible vascular injuries or obvious compartment syndrome.

The presence of concomitant diseases, such as diabetes or peripheral vascular disease, must also be considered, as they can worsen local conditions or have negative post-operative effects on the operation site or significantly increase the risk of onset of the complications of deep infection. Not infrequently in such patients oedema, superficial blisters or simple skin abrasion can transform a closed injury into an open injury through the loss of skin substance [6].

Treatment Options

There are at least three surgical options reported frequently in the literature for the treatment of these types of injuries and they differ on the type of fixator used, the timing of the treatment and lastly the surgical technique employed.

1. *Complete internal osteosynthesis* after Open Reduction and Internal Fixation (ORIF) is generally preferred in low-energy injuries with soft tissue damage not greater than Tscheme Grade I.

    This treatment, according to AO principles, provides for:
- open reduction and synthesis of the fibula to restore bone length using a direct lateral surgical approach;
- reconstruction of the articular surface with temporary stabilisation of bone fragments using K-wires, accessing via an anterior distal tibial approach;
- bone graft in the metaphyseal area when necessary;
- synthesis using a plate and screws via an anterior or medial approach, possibly with limited surgical access (Fig. 3) [7].
2. *Minimal internal osteosynthesis* of the epiphyseal region associated with stabilisation with an external fixator is preferable in injuries with severe soft tissue damage (Tscherne Grades II and III) [7]. In these cases, if the main area of comminution is in the metaphysis, the fracture site can be stabilised using a hybrid or circular monosegmental fixator. If there is epiphyseal comminution, the use of a bridging fixator is recommended.

When an articulated fixator is used, early joint movement can be anticipated without the need to exchange fixators [4]. Alternatively, a static bridging fixator can be exchanged for a monosegmental fixator at the appropriate time after application.

3. Minimal internal epiphyseal osteosynthesis in conjunction with a *temporary external fixator* that allows for soft tissue healing and subsequent definitive internal synthesis is one of the options used by some Authors in injuries of Tscherne Grades II and III or Ruedi and Allgower Types II and III, as an alternative to an articulated or hybrid external fixator. This approach has the advantages of allowing rapid recovery of articulation and

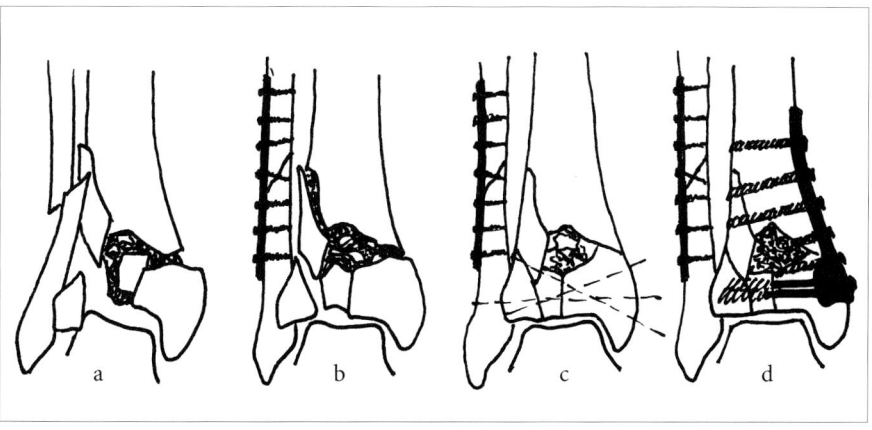

Fig. 3. *AO criteria for definitive internal fixation (ORIF) in tibial pilon injuries.* **a** Pre-operative planning. **b** Fibular fixation. **c** Minimal internal fixation of the epiphyseal region. **d** Extensive fixation of the distal tibia with a medial plate and screws and bone grafting of the the metaphysis

guaranteeing sufficient metaphyseal stability, although there is a degree of risk regarding complications connected with ORIF surgery [3, 7-9].

There are two alternative treatment options that provide for:

- conservative treatment using plaster cast and calcaneal traction wires. This regime is reserved for patients with open injuries (Ruedi and Allgower Type I) and patients in serious overall condition;
- surgical treatment by immediate arthrodesis using an external fixator, plate or retrograde intramedullary screws or nail. This treatment is used exclusively on patients with Type III injuries and limited functional requirements.

Current Trends

Reduction of the fracture and reconstruction of the articular surface are the critical part of surgery, especially where there is comminution.

Following recent reports in the literature, definitive internal fixation is no longer used to repair tibial pilon fractures, due to the high risk of complications and great reliability of current, less invasive techniques [10].

External fixation in combination with minimal internal fixation has been shown to be the best surgical solution for these injuries, as it guarantees stability and respects the biological processes at the fracture site. The design of frame and fixation to be used is determined by the fracture type, particularly whether the injury belongs to the *simple articular injury* category (Ruedi and

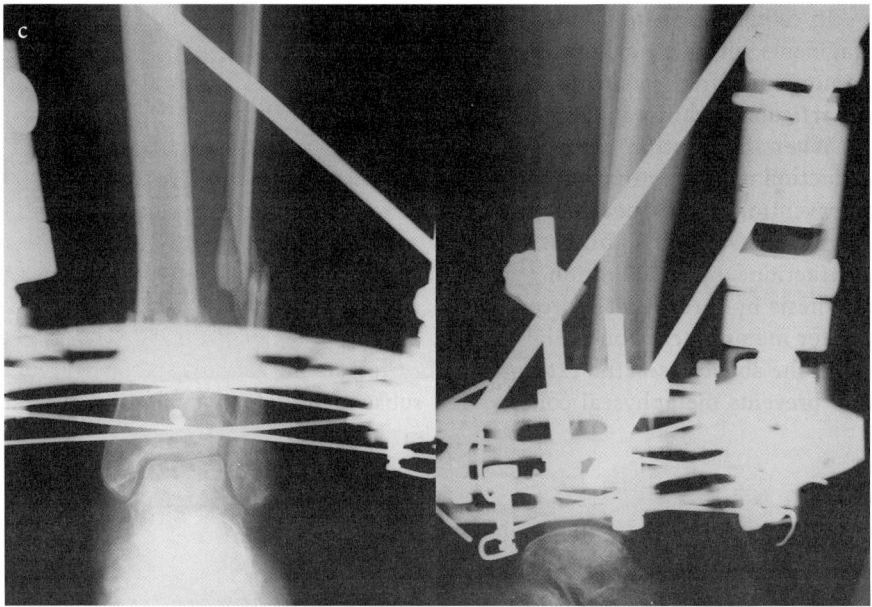

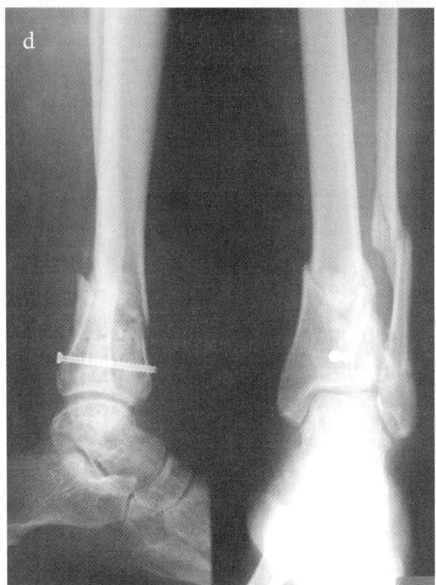

Fig. 6. c X-Rays at external fixator removal (16 weeks), and at follow-up (2 years) (**d**)

also reduces the incidence of tissue necrosis and deep infection. An articulated fixator permits early mobilisation and encourages functional tibio-tarsal recovery. It also permits partial, often early weightbearing, which may be fundamental in stimulating bone repair and in preventing algodystrophy.

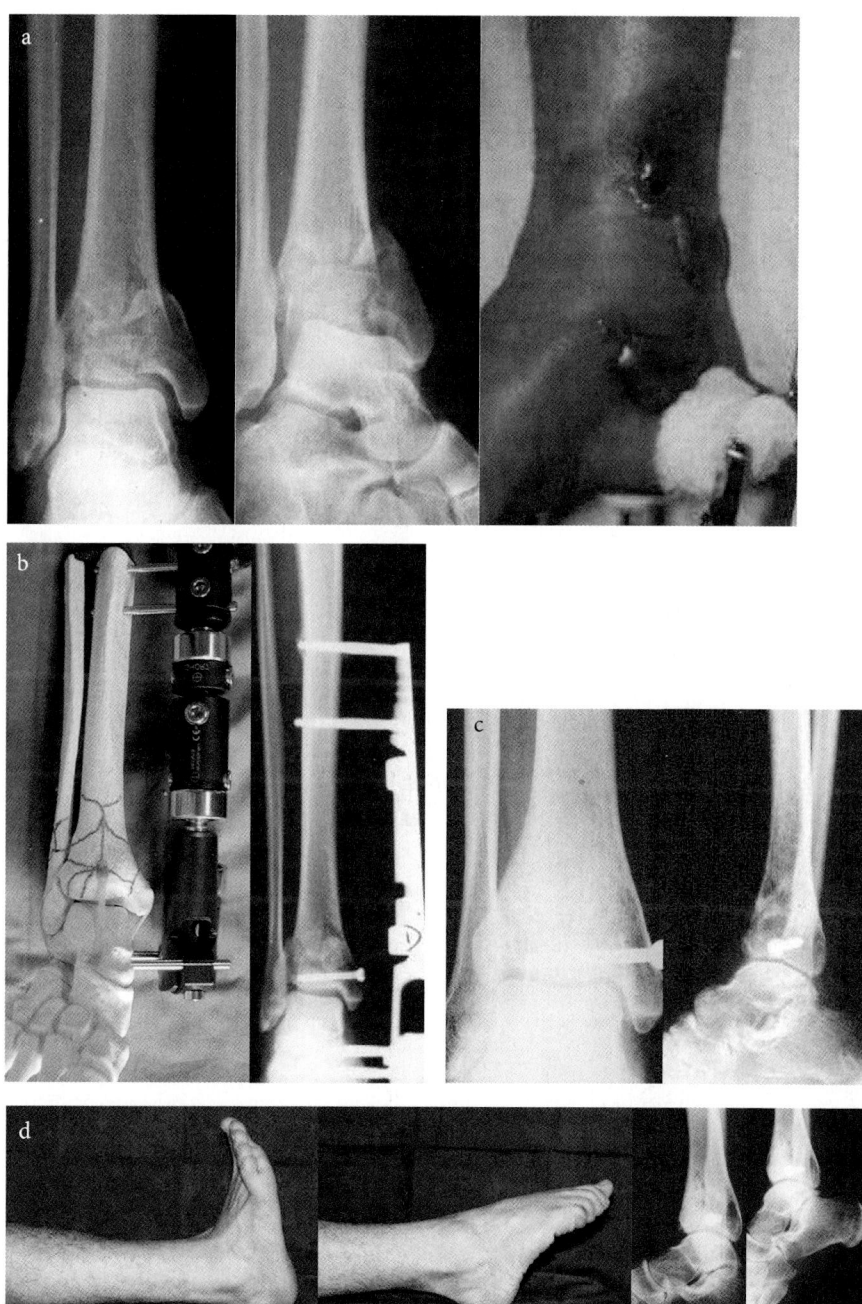

Fig. 7. a Complex articular fracture with epiphyseal comminution and severe soft tissue damage Tscherne Grade II. **b** Stabilisation in distraction with ligamentotaxis and cutaneous synthesis. **c** X-Ray check when healed (12 weeks). **d** Clinical and X-Ray checks at follow-up (4 years)

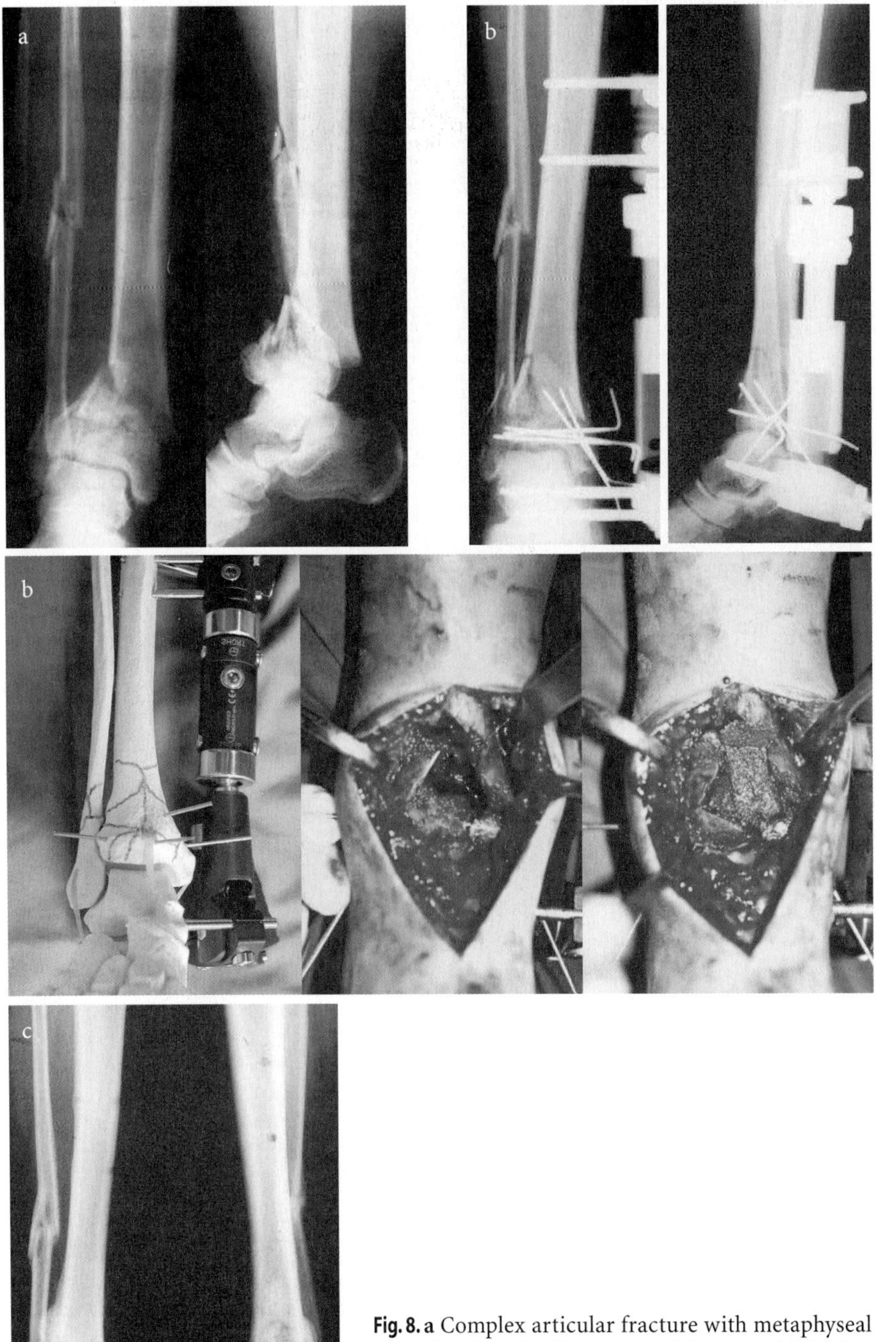

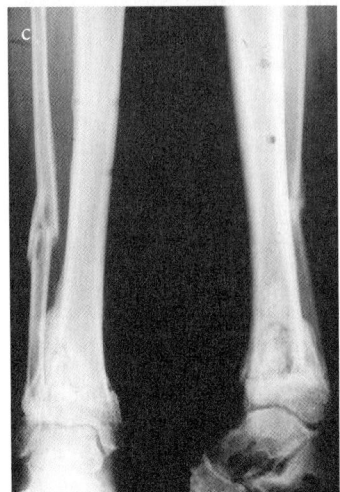

Fig. 8. a Complex articular fracture with metaphyseal comminution. **b** Treatment with external bridging fixator in distraction in combination with open reduction and minimal internal fixation with K-wires. The loss of metaphyseal substance is treated with cancellous bone graft. **c** X-Ray at follow-up (6 months)

Additional Surgery

Presuming that external fixation provides correct axial alignment and length, anatomic fibular synthesis is not obligatory and can in fact hinder healing of the tibial injury. On the other hand, fibular synthesis is recommended where there is a complete injury with distal tibio-fibular syndesmosis. As previously mentioned, bone grafting is carried out in all cases of severe loss of metaphyseal substance after open reduction of the articular fracture. Deferred bone graft is very rarely required after closed ligamentotaxis.

References

1. Geissler WB, Tsao AK, Hughes JL (1996) Fractures and injuries of the ankle. In: Rockwood CA Jr, Green DP (eds) Fractures in adults, Vol. 2, 4th edn. Lippincott-Raven, Philadelphia New York, pp 2236-2242
2. Whittle AP (1998) Fractures of lower extremity. In: Canale ST (ed) Campbell's operative orthopaedics, Vol. 3, 9th edn. Mosby, St. Louis, pp 2057-2066
3. Borrelli J Jr, Ellis E (2002) Pilon fractures: assessment and treatment. Orthop Clin North Am 33(1):231-245
4. Renzi Brivio L, Lavini F, Cavina Pratesi F et al (2000) L'uso della fissazione esterna nelle fratture del pilone tibiale. Chir Org Mov 85(3):205-214
5. Sirkin M, Sanders R (2001) The treatment of pilon fractures. Orthop Clin North Am 32(1):91-102
6. Watson JT, Moed BR, Karges DE, Cramer KE (2000) Pilon fractures. Treatment protocol based on severity of soft tissue injury. Clin Orthop (375):78-90
7. Blauth M, Bastian L, Krettek C et al (2001) Surgical options for the treatment of severe tibial pilon fractures: a study of three techniques. J Orthop Trauma 15(3):153-160
8. Patterson M, Cole J (1999) Two staged delayed open reduction and internal fixation of severe pilon tibial fractures. J Orthop Trauma 13(2):85-91
9. Thordarson DB (2000) Complications after treatment of tibial pilon fractures: prevention and management strategies. J Am Acad Orthop Surg 8(4):253-265
10. Sirkin M, Sanders R, Di Pasquale T, Herscovici D Jr (1999) A staged protocol for soft tissue management in the treatment of complex pilon fractures. J Orthop Trauma 13(2):78-84

Conservative Treatment: How and When?

F. Biggi, A. Cipriano, G. Costacurta, C. Gios, E. Scalco

Introduction

The standard term *tibial pilon fracture* is used for a group of injuries of the most distal part of the tibia, either intra or extra-capsular. There is almost always involvement of the articular surface which represents the dome of the tibio-fibulo-talar joint complex. Tibial pilon fractures comprise approximately 7% of tibial fractures and 1% of lower limb fractures but have always been a major problem in traumatology. The fractures are frequently comminuted with soft tissue damage and this makes the choice of therapy more difficult. This is the type of situation seen more often in modern practice with an increase in high-energy trauma events following workplace and road traffic accidents. When the force is directed vertically (fall injuries to the heels, frontal car crashes), the distal articular surface of the tibia can give way with varying degrees of comminution and/or depression.

On the other hand, in low energy trauma, for example in skiing or contact sports, fractures tend to be oblique or less displaced [1, 2]. The talus is almost always displaced in these types of injury and it is worth emphasising that reduction is the key treatment. It can restore length to the damaged bone segment and correct the tension in the ligament-capsule complex. Another characteristic of these fractures is that the mean patient age is 35-40. Clearly unsuitable treatment will have consequences leading to invalidity, and complications can arise even after a "successful" operation [3-5].

It is widely held in traumatology that anatomical reduction of the articular surface should be achieved, as far as possible, in these types of fractures, to provide long-term stability and more rapid return to joint mobility.

The complications resulting from different types of treatment are self evident, particularly in open fractures, such as infection, poor consolidation, non union and degenerative arthropathy [6-8].

UOA di Ortopedia e Traumatologia, USSL 3, Asiago

Conservative Treatment

Modern traumatology is now rejecting conservative treatment based on the application of plastercasts. This trend is apparent given the diversity of internal and external osteosynthesis now available. They have put an end to "fracture illness", the direct result of long periods of immobilisation.

Industry and surgeons working together have developed techniques and instruments that can guarantee fracture reduction, immediate and long-term stability, rapid return to mobility and a more rapid return to the patient's daily life.

Is there still any need for conservative treatment? We believe that there are currently two types of fracture that may benefit from this option: 1) displaced or slightly displaced fractures; 2) fractures with soft tissue damage requiring deferment of final treatment.

Displaced or Slightly Displaced Fractures

When planning the type of treatment, whether surgical or non-surgical, it is good practice to consider the classification of the injury. This will identify the varying degrees of fragmentation and stage the different phases of treatment from casualty admission through to the operating theatre. There are various classifications for this type of fracture [1, 4, 8]: as there is an increasing tendency towards international uniformity of the language of traumatology, we feel that the "AO Classification" proposed by Müller, Nazarian and Koch should be adopted. This system places injuries in three main groups: a) extra-articular, b) partial articular, c) complete articular. There are three progressive subgroups relative to prognostic severity and subsequent treatment difficulties.

Diagnosis is mainly by radiography, and standard antero-posterior, lateral and oblique views are often sufficient. Either 2D or 3D CT is invaluable in cases of widespread comminution for planning reconstruction and, if necessary, for evaluating any requirement for internal fixation, especially when comminution is associated with crushing of the trabeculae in cancellous bone.

Only displaced fractures where there is an articular gap not more than 1 mm are suited to conservative treatment, and this is only applicable to young patients, who are under 60, active and have a life expectancy of at least another 20 years.

Conservative treatment may also be appropriate where there are other biological factors such as diabetes, lower-limb vasculopathy, decubitus ulcers, neoplasms with poor life expectancy and significant local or systemic infection.

Conservative treatment is based on a traditional plastercast preceded possibly by transcalcaneal wire traction, and aims to achieve the best alignment possible and a reduction in the swelling usually associated with these types of injuries. The plastercast (or other material) will initially be long leg, enabling the patient to walk with the help of forearm-crutches. The knee is flexed at 30°

inside the cast, with the ankle in slight equinus to avoid any diastasis of the tibio-fibular syndesmosis caused by the talus, which widens with dorsiflexion of the foot. The full leg cast allows fibro-cartilage to form and stabilise the fracture fragments, and can be replaced after about three weeks and with a standard below knee walking cast to allow weightbearing for about five weeks.

One radiographic check is sufficient after applying the below knee cast. Other X-Rays may be made for reasons of accident insurance claims or at the onset of any local symptoms. Physiotherapy should begin immediately the cast is removed, and should include ankle mobilisation, isometric muscular strengthening of the lower limb, proprioceptive exercises and walking with a correct gait.

Soft Tissue Damage

Soft tissue damage and other possible injuries (fractures of the calcaneus, talus, tibial shaft, pelvis and vertebrae) are frequently associated with these types of lesion and the worse the skeletal involvement, the worse the overall trauma.

When the joint is being examined, particular attention should be paid to the neurovascular status, bruising, tissue tension, the appearance of blisters and potential avascular areas where skin necrosis may occur. Observation of these patients is therefore very important in the period after hospital admission and it should be noted that urgent treatment, whether conservative or surgical, is not always the best course [1, 2, 6].

When there is significant soft tissue damage with even minimal fracture displacement, it may be preferable to apply transcalcaneal traction, thus ensuring complete visibility of the segment, and enabling continued wound toilet, medication and more effective pain control. If the pain is severe, a decision should be made about the most appropriate treatment, while the patient is provided with antithrombotic and antibiotic cover.

Transcalcaneal traction may also be valuable for definitive treatment, whether conservative or possibly surgical, as it provides control during reduction manoeuvres and adds further stability if incorporated in a cast.

Conclusions

Conservative treatment would seem to have an increasingly limited role to play in the treatment of tibial-pilon fractures which require anatomical reduction, appropriate stabilisation and mobilisation as soon as possible [1, 4, 7, 8].

The possible immediate and long-term complications of surgery are well described and may be independent of the techniques used. These high energy trauma events almost always involve damage to the ankle articular surfaces with significant displacement and comminution. These injuries usually require a surgically proactive, approach, and there are few cases which can be treated

of these is that of Ruedi and Allgower [9-11], based on analysis of comminution and displacement of articular fragmentation (Fig. 1).

This classification has two significant advantages: it is very easy to apply in the practical sense and it is unparalleled as a prognostic tool, as will be seen in our study.

In the past, there was an argument that conservative treatment for complex tibial pilon fractures was preferable, given the high risk of secondary complications from surgery and the difficulty in obtaining stable synthesis. Today it is agreed that the best results for displaced tibial pilon fractures, as in other articular fractures, are obtained when anatomical reduction and synthesis are combined so as to give a rapid return to normal functioning [7, 9, 10, 12].

Healed fractures with articular irregularities and interfragmentary gaps of more than 2 mm are considered therapeutic failures, as they will inevitably

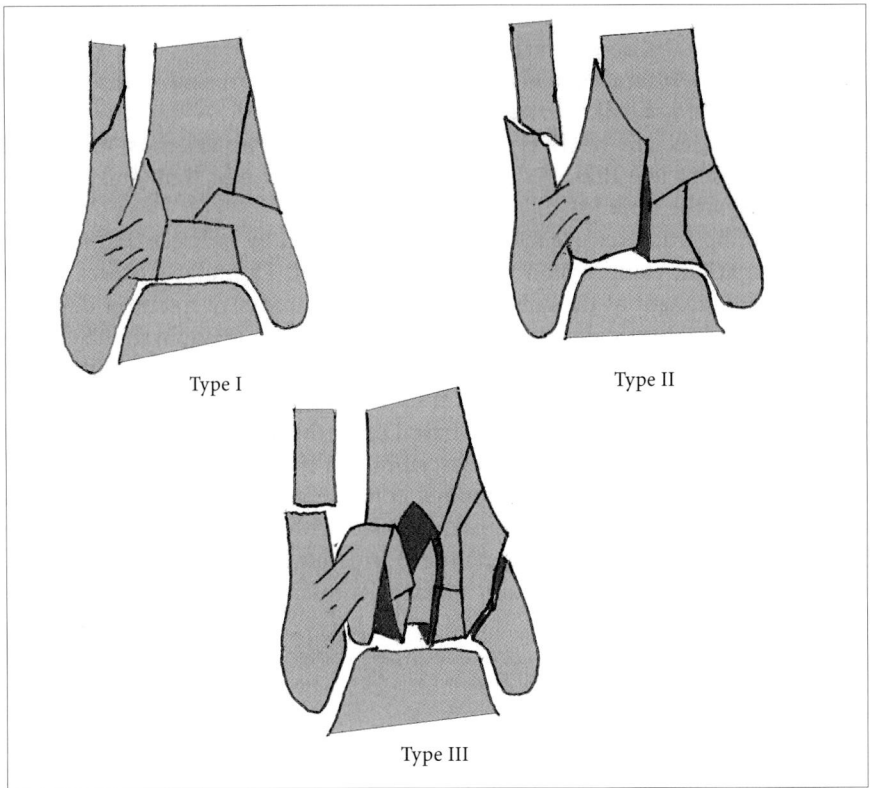

Fig. 1. The Ruedi and Allgower Classification. *Type 1:* "cleavage-type" fracture with no comminution or articular fragment displacement. *Type II:* "cleavage-type" fracture with minimal comminution, but with articular fracture-line displacement. *Type III:* displaced and comminuted fracture

evolve into a highly symptomatic post-traumatic arthrosis that will require further surgery, such as tibio-tarsal arthrodesis or ankle prosthesis.

Even a correctly conducted operation in this particular area runs a significant risk of complications, which usually stem from soft tissue problems (skin necrosis, infection after wound dehiscence, loss of reduction leading to infection). In view of these potential problems in dealing with high-energy, severely comminuted fractures complicated by significant soft tissue damage, opinion has changed in recent times to favour less invasive, more "biological" surgery using minimal internal osteosynthesis in association with ligamentotaxis and external fixation [13-15].

This study aims to achieve two different objectives: to pool the thoughts and ideas of those who treat fractures of this type to draw up a standard method of treatment; and to verify the proposed model through critical analysis with a view to establishing guidelines regarding morphological treatment, relating this to the severity of soft tissue damage and the recommended choice of therapy.

Materials and Methods

The sample population consisted of 42 patients, 24 males (57.1%) and 18 females (42.9%) treated between 1994-1998 at the Department of Orthopaedics and Traumatology of the G. Pini Orthopaedic Institute in Milan.

Two of the patients had bilateral injuries and of the others 66.7% had injuries to the left side. Mean age was 45 years and 6 months (range 16-73 years) and the accident circumstances are listed in Table 1.

The most common skeletal injury was ipsilateral fracture of the fibula (68.2%).

Using the Ruedi and Allgower classification, the fractures were sub-divided as follows: 31.8% were Type I, 22.7% were Type II and 45.5% were Type III. Eight of the fractures (18.2%) were open.

Table 1. Accident circumstances

Falls from a height	33.3%
Other falls (in or out of home)	33.3%
Road traffic accidents	9.6%
Sports accidents (skiing, football, ice-hockey)	23.8%

The chosen treatment was rigid internal fixation in 90.9% of cases and external fixation in 9.1%. Further surgery was required in 27.3% of cases. An equal number of the fractures required plastic-reconstructive surgery.

Mean follow-up period was 4.3 years (range 2.5–6.2 years) The long time span between injury and final evaluation was deliberate so as not to exclude any possible dysfunction from secondary arthrosis. Complications of this type can generally be identified by radiography within the first post-operative year and in the Authors' view identification all cases of secondary degenerative arthropathy is reliable after a two year interval [9-11].

Treatment

Accurate reduction with solid fixation permits fragment reduction under direct vision. Stable synthesis cannot be obtained by open surgery which exposes the fracture site [16].

The following are the goals in all cases:
1. a minimally invasive surgical approach that takes vascularisation into account;
2. anatomical reduction;
3. stable osteosynthesis;
4. early mobilisation.

These four objectives must always be considered during surgical planning, which is of equal importance to the surgery itself. The fundamentals of planning are as follows:
1. the timing of surgery: as oedema appears 8-12 hours after the trauma event and generally doesn't resolve before 7-10 days, it is essential not to intervene during this time span in which the risk of causing complications is at its highest;
2. selecting the surgical approach: antero-medial access is almost always the most convenient route but consideration of the fracture morphology may result in less conventional approaches being preferable, such as antero-lateral or posterior;
3. evaluation of the tibio-fibular lateral wall: the majority of injury patterns included fibular fractures which required treatment to restore correct leg length and avoid the onset of valgus malunion;
4. anticipating results of reduction: if the syndesmosis is complete, as in the majority of cases, the Tillaux-Chaput tubercle and surgically fixed fibula unite to provide a surgical platform for the alignment of the remaining large fragments. The smaller fragments simply adapt to the shape of the talar dome. Should this not occur, reduction can become considerably more complicated and can only be achieved through ligamentotaxis;
5. choice of implant: if the bone stock is suitable and there is no severe comminution, we believe that interfragmentary screws are sufficient. Failing this, a support plate is indispensable (Fig. 2);

6. the use of preferably autologous cortico-cancellous bone graft where there is a significant defect of the metaphyseal area.

The antero-medial approach has the advantage of respecting the soft tissue vascular supply [17], and interferes with only the anterior tibial artery, leaving the peroneal and posterior tibial arteries untouched (Fig. 3). With the aim of maintaining adequate cutaneous vascularisation, it is further recommended that there is at least 7-8 cm between incisions over the tibial and fibular sites [3].

Although the literature recommends various types of implant, our experience relates mostly to the cloverleaf and spoon plates. We have found the cloverleaf to be particularly useful because of its ease of adaptability to the tibial epiphysis and if necessary, including the medial malleolus.

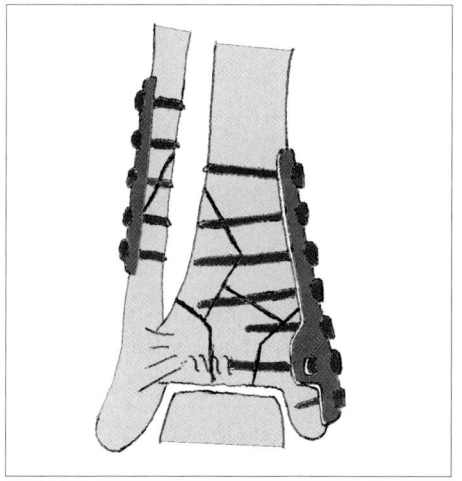

Fig. 2. Osteosynthesis of the distal tibial metaphysis with medial support plate and fibular malleolus with 1/3 tubular plate

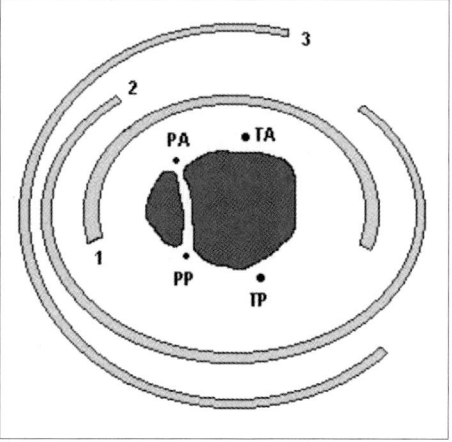

Fig. 3. Areas of vascularisation. *1:* anterior tibial artery *(TA)*. *2:* posterior tibial artery *(TP)*. *3:* anterior *(PA)* and posterior peroneal arteries *(PP)*

Although the plate tends to be medially positioned to prevent varus displacement, sometimes the direction of the fracture-line requires fixation on the antero-medial surface (Figs. 4, 5).

We are of the opinion that external fixation offers a valid alternative to internal synthesis only in certain circumstances:
- open fractures;
- closed fractures with severe soft tissue damage;
- highly comminuted fractures;
- polytrauma.

Transarticular fixation [18, 19] is the means of first choice in cases of severe articular comminution as ligamentotaxis provides satisfactory reduction with the absence of sites suitable for fixation in the epiphysis.

This technique is often completed by surgical reduction and minimally invasive fixation with K-wires or screws.

We fix a fibular fracture prior to applying external fixation (Fig. 6).

We have found it useful to exchange the bridging fixation for hybrid fixation with distal tibial rings after 30 days to allow early ankle mobilisation.

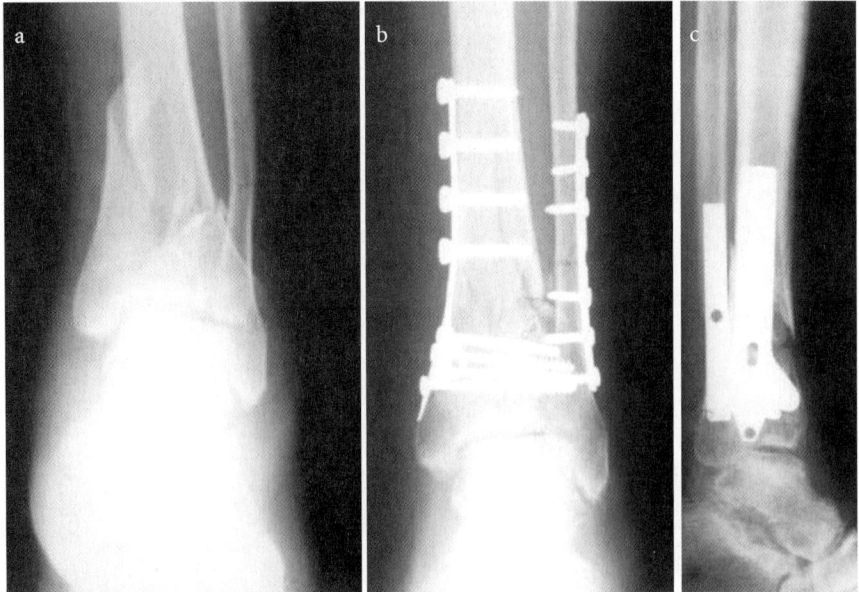

Fig. 4. *38 year-old female. Closed Type II Ruedi and Allgower fracture.* **a** Pre-operative X-Ray. **b, c** Post-operative check after 4 years, result judged as "excellent"

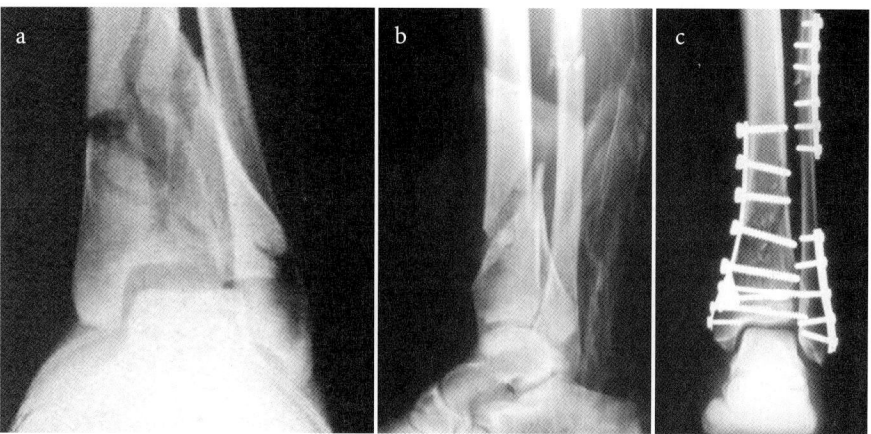

Fig. 5. *54 year-old female. Closed Type II fracture associated with bifocal fibular fracture.* **a, b** Pre-operative X-Rays. **c** Post-operative X-Rays after 5 years. The result objectively and subjectively is "good"

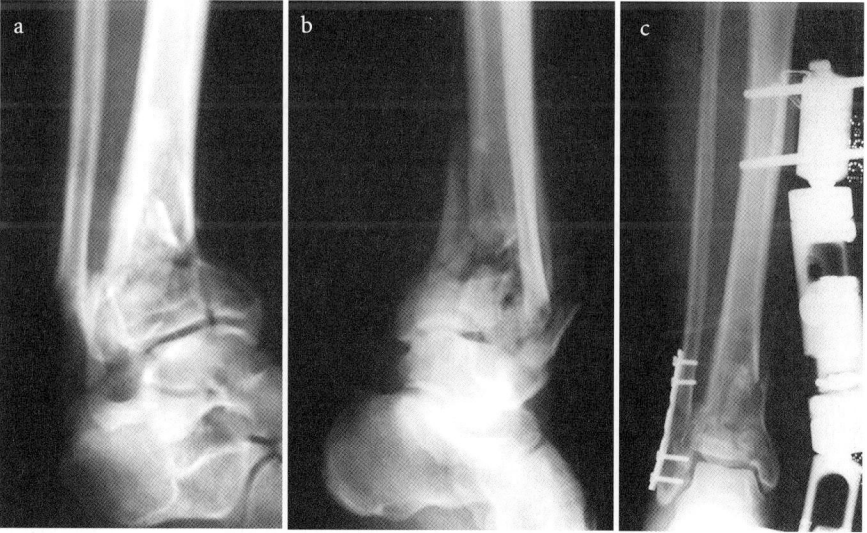

Fig. 6. *31 year-old male. Closed Type III Ruedi and Allgower fracture.* **a, b** Pre-operative X-Rays severe varus displacement. **c** Post-operative X-Rays. Stabilisation with external Orthofix fixator in transarticular bridging. After 3 years. Result objectively judged "good" and subjectively "fair"

Results

There is a lack of agreement between Authors on the methodology of of evaluating the results of treatment [7, 12, 20, 21].

The Ovadia and Beals system [7] would seem to be least liable to error and subjective misinterpretation.

The results are expressed by three criteria, good, fair or poor, and these are assessed objectively and subjectively. Tables 2 and 3 show the evaluation results. Final outcome irrespective of injury severity is shown in Tables 4 and 5.

If the fractures are classified according to Ruedi and Allgower, the categories tend to be uniform in their degree of severity.

Type I fractures (31.8%; 14 patients) had results shown in Table 6. Internal synthesis was the method used in 85.7% and external fixation in the remaining 2 cases (14.3%). The 10 (22.7%) Type II cases were treated by internal fixation, with the results shown in Table 7.

Table 2. Objective evaluation of results according to Ovadia and Beals [7]

| Parameters | Criteria | | | |
	Excellent	Good	Fair	Poor
ROM	> 75%	50-75%	25-50%	< 25%
T-T alignment	in axis	in axis	< 5°	> 5°
Tibial shortening	absent	absent	< 1 cm	> 1 cm
Chronic oedema	absent	slight	moderate	severe
Prone supination	normal	normal	slightly reduced	very reduced
Fixed deformity	absent	absent	absent	present

Table 3. Subjective evalution of results according to Ovadia and Beals [7]

| Parameters | Criteria | | | |
	Excellent	Good	Fair	Poor
Pain	absent	slight	moderate	severe
Return to work	same job	same job	different job	impossible
Recreational activity	unchanged	slightly changed	greatly changed	impossible
Limitations to walking	absent	absent	present	present
Analgesics	not necessary	not necessary	necessary	opiates
Limp	absent	absent	occasional	persistent

Table 4. Overall objective results – Ovadia and Beals

Excellent	50%
Good	30%
Fair	10%
Poor	10%

Table 5. Overall subjective results – Ovadia and Beals

Excellent	31.8%
Good	36.4%
Fair	27.3%
Poor	4.5%

Table 6. Results for Type I fractures

Result	Objective	Subjective
Excellent	75%	28.6%
Good	25%	57.1%
Fair	0	14.3%
Poor	0	0

Table 7. Results for Type II fractures

Result	Objective	Subjective
Excellent	100%	60%
Good	0	20%
Fair	0	20%
Poor	0	0

Type III fractures (45.5%; 20 patients) were treated primarily with internal fixation in 90% of cases and with an external fixator in the remaining 10% (2 patients). The results are shown in Table 8.

Sixteen out of 44 or 36.4% of the cases studied had complications (Table 9). The sum of percentages is more than 36.4% as some patients had more than one complication.

Two of the 8 confirmed deep infections occurred in open fractures and four in fractures associated with soft tissue compromise. The exact cause in the remaining 2 cases was probably related to over-aggressive internal fixation.

When infection occurred, targeted antibiotics were used based on the results of culture and sensitivity; the fixation method was changed from internal to external fixation in four cases, and, where required by soft tissue debridement, with a subsequent operation to provide skin cover. Excellent

Often, all this is not possible in a single operation, and perhaps it is better to describe a surgical process rather than a single operation, and think of it as a dynamic multi-step approach to tibial pilon fractures. External fixation applied as a matter of urgency could perhaps be advantageously changed for internal synthesis (on the advice of a plastic surgeon), when the skin situation is more favourable. There are also many other possible treatments including the use of hybrid fixation to be considered.

All things considered, we feel that an approach to tibial pilon fractures that abandons traditional preconceptions and takes a more multi-disciplinary and dynamic attitude, while not being the easiest option, undoubtedly offers the best guarantee of a successful outcome for the patient.

Acknowledgements: The Authors would like to thank Luisella Meloni for her work in drawing up this document.

References

1. Destot E (1911) Traumatismes du pied et rayons x malleoles, astragale, calcaneum, avant-pied. Masson, Paris
2. Bonin JG (1950) Injuries to the ankle. William Heinemann, London
3. Helfet DL, Koval K, Pappas J et al (1994) Intraarticular "pilon" fracture of the tibia. Clin Orthop 298:221-228
4. Kellam JF, Waddell JP (1979) Fractures of the distal tibial metaphysis with intra-articular extension: the distal tibial explosion fracture. J Trauma 19(8):593-601
5. Lauge-Hansen N (1953) Fractures of the ankle V: pronation-dorsiflexion fractures. Arch Surg 67:813-820
6. Maale G, Seligson D (1980) Fractures through the weightbearing surface of the distal tibia. Orthopedics 3:517-521
7. Ovadia DN, Beals RK (1986) Fractures of the tibial plafond. J Bone Joint Surg Am 68(4):543-551
8. Vives P, Hourlier H, De Lestang M et al (1984) Etude de 84 fractures du pilon tibial de l'adulte. Essay de classification. Rev Chir Ortop 70(2):129-139
9. Ruedi TP, Allgower M (1969) Fractures of the lower end of the tibia into the ankle joint. Injury 1:92-99
10. Ruedi TP (1973) Fractures of the lower end of the tibia into the ankle joint: results nine years after open reduction and internal fixation. Injury 5:130-134
11. Ruedi TP, Allgower M (1979) The operative treatment of intra-articular fractures of the lower end of the tibia. Clin Orthop (138):105-110
12. Burwell HN, Charnley AD (1965) The treatment of displaced fractures of the ankle by rigid internal fixation and early joint movement. J Bone Joint Surg Br 47(4):634-660
13. Bone L, Stegemann P, McNamara K, Seibel R (1993) External fixation of severely comminuted and open tibial pilon fractures. Clin Orthop (292):101-107
14. Pugh KJ, Wolinsky PR, McAndrew MP, Johnson KD (1999) Tibial pilon fractures: a comparison of treatment methods. J Trauma 47(5):937-941
15. Saleh M, Shanahan G, Fern ED (1993) Intra-articular fractures of the distal tibia : surgical management by minimal internal fixation and articulated distraction. Injury 24(1):37-40

16. Ruedi TP, Murphy WL (2000) AO principles of fracture management, Chapt. 4.8.3. AO Publishing, Thieme

17. Bour P, Aubry P, Fieve G (1992) Vascularisation du pilon tibial: applications thèrapeutiques. 66° Réunion annuelle de la SOFCOT Les fractures récentes du pilon tibial de l'adulte. Rev Chir Orthop 78[Suppl 1]:47-48

18. Marsh JL, Lavini F: Distal tibial and pilon fractures. Operative technique. Orthofix Operative Technique Manual n.7. In: www.orthofix.com

19. Treadwell JR, Fallat LM (1994) Dynamic unilateral distraction fixation: surgical management of tibial pilon fractures. J Foot Ankle Surg 33(5):438-442

20. Gaudinez RF, Mallik AR, Szporn M (1996) Hybrid external fixation in tibial plafond fractures. Clin Orthop 329:223-232

21. Marsh JL, Bonar S, Nepola JV et al (1995) Use of an articulated external fixator for fractures of the tibial plafond. J Bone Joint Surg Am 77(10):1498-1509

22. Babis GC, Vayanos ED, Papaioannou N (1997) Pantazopoulos T: results of surgical treatment of tibial plafond fractures. Clin Orthop (341):99-105

23. Barbieri R, Schenk R, Koval K et al (1996) Hybrid external fixation in the treatment of tibial plafond fractures. Clin Orthop (332):16-22

24. Gustilo RB (1989) Management of open fractures. In: Gustilo RB (ed) Orthopaedic infection: diagnosis and treatment. WB Saunders, Philadelphia, pp 87-117

Treatment with External Fixation

M. Manca[1], F. Lavini[2]

External fixation was initially used as a first aid treatment, often temporary, for fractures which were severely open or associated with polytrauma [1]. More recently it has been used by some authors as the method of choice in complex fractures of the tibial pilon, and the technique has been steadily gaining in popularity [2-5].

The preference that surgeons have for this technique is founded on the decreased incidence of short and mid-term complications (osteomyelitis, deep infection and non union) compared to Open Reduction and Internal Fixation (ORIF) with screws and plates. It is not related to improved long-term results, for which the two methods seem to be equivalent [6-8].

External fixation provides the advantage that the metaphyseal portion of these fractures can be stabilised without using an internal subcutaneous implant [6]. External fixation, whether with screws or tensioned wires, is generally tolerated well round the hind-foot and ankle.

The results and techniques of three external fixation methods have been described in the literature [6, 9]:

1. a frame consisting of a hybrid fixator with a ring supporting periarticular distal tibial tensioned wires (Fig. 1);
2. an ankle bridging fixator that does not permit any movement (Fig. 2);
3. an ankle bridging fixator that permits a certain degree of movement at the tibio-tarsal joint (Fig. 3).

Currently there is insufficient experience or bibliographic data to determine the advantages, disadvantages, and long-term results of each method.

[1] I Clinica Ortopedica di Pisa, [2] Clinica Ortopedica di Verona

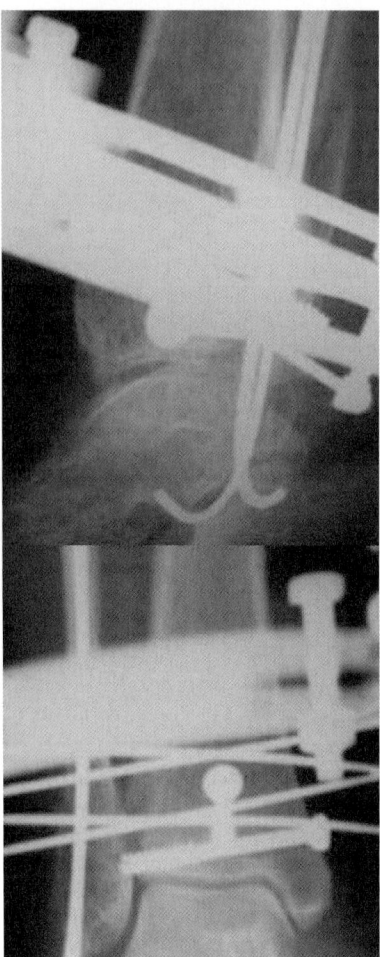

Fig. 1. X-Ray of a fracture with screws in the epiphysis and a ring with tensioned wires on the metaphysis

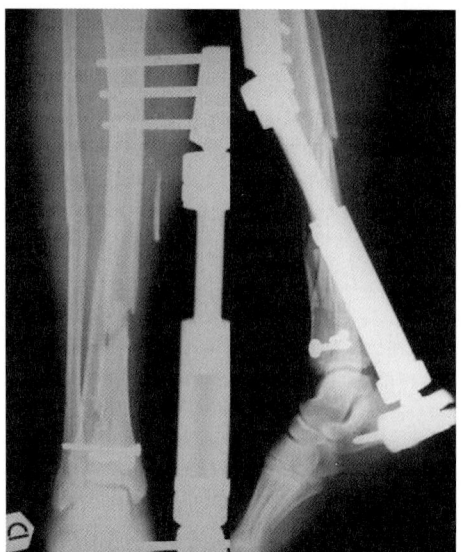

Fig. 2. An external bridging ankle fixator which is not articulated

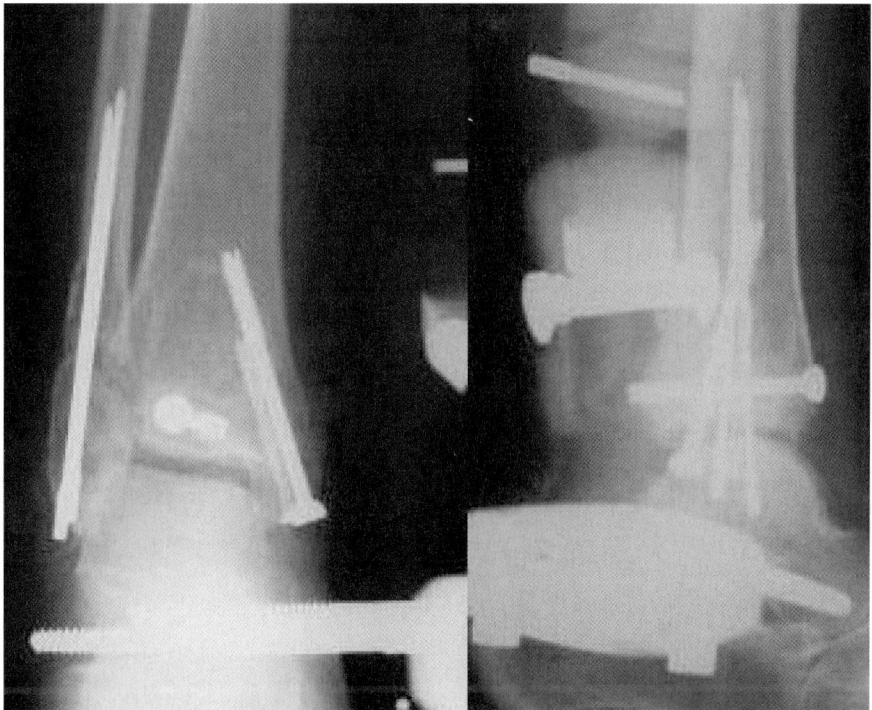

Fig. 3. An articulated external bridging ankle fixator

However, it has been clearly demonstrated that use of an external fixator in high-energy complex fractures of the tibial pilon will reduce the early complication rate [4, 8].

Regarding the AO classification [7], treatment with an external fixator is described for Type A fractures, i.e. in distal extra-articular fractures that may have a simple fracture line in the metaphyseal area (Type A1), a cuneiform comminuted fracture (Type A2) or a complex metaphyseal comminution (Type A3).

External fixation may also be indicated in some Type B fractures with partial articular involvement, particularly those with articular comminution.

Almost always, treatment with external fixation can be used for the more serious Type C fractures, and is usually combined with internal fixation of the articular surface, whether C1, uncomminuted, C2 with metaphyseal but no articular comminution, or C3 with articular and metaphyseal comminution.

Description of the Various Types of Assembly

A Hybrid Fixator with Tensioned Wires just Proximal to the Tibiotarsal Joint

Assembly of a hybrid implant requires a ring with tensioned wires on the tibial epiphysis attached to a fixator body and reinforced with bars in different planes to ensure stability by neutralising the bending loads (Fig. 4).

This assembly is mono-segmental and does not bridge the joint, permitting passive and active articular movement from the beginning.

The rings can be complete or two thirds.

The first step is restoration of fibular length, if indicated.

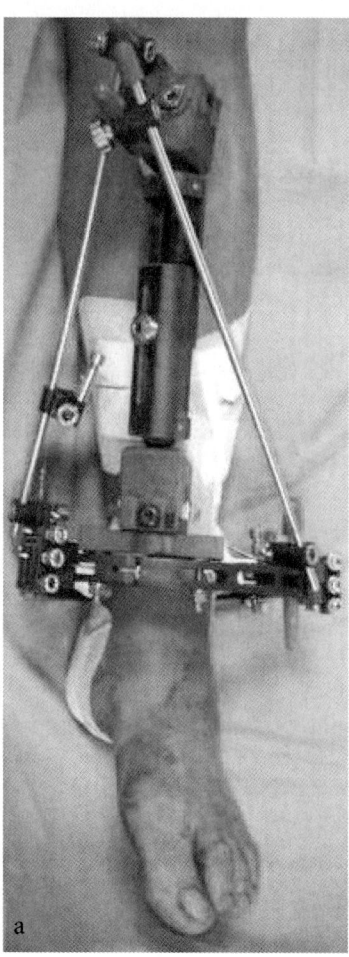
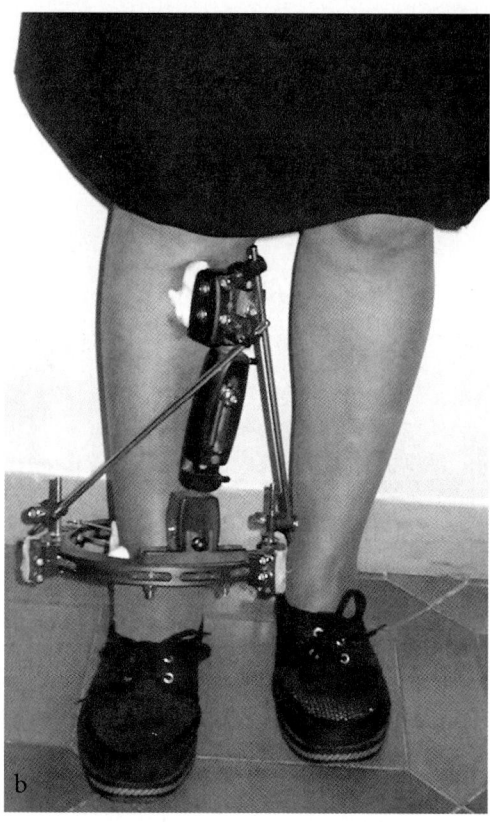

Fig. 4. *Examples of hybrid fixation with reinforcing bars.* **a** Immediately post-operatively. **b** While weight-bearing

This can be performed with intramedullary rods through the lateral malleolus, when the fibula fracture is short transverse or oblique.

If the fracture is comminuted or long oblique, open fixation with plate and screws is advisable.

The next step is always to reduce the tibial articular surface, by closed manipulation if possible.

To improve the pre-operative planning, and to enable reduction manoeuvres to be performed closed when possible, a CT study of the fracture, possibly with two-dimensional reconstruction, is very helpful.

The limb is positioned on the traction bed with transcalcaneal traction.

Closed reduction, when possible, can be carried out with reduction forceps or by introducing K-wires into the epiphyseal fragments under X-Ray control, and moving them like joysticks to reduce the fragments. K-wires are advanced and used as guide wires for cannulated screws to provide internal fixation (Fig. 5).

In other cases, when the fragments are more central and cannot be reached directly with transcortical wires, a small incision is made over the medial face of the tibia proximally, above the metaphyseal fracture [10].

A small window is made with a 4.8-mm drill.

A suitably shaped K-wire is inserted to push the articular fragment down from the inside.

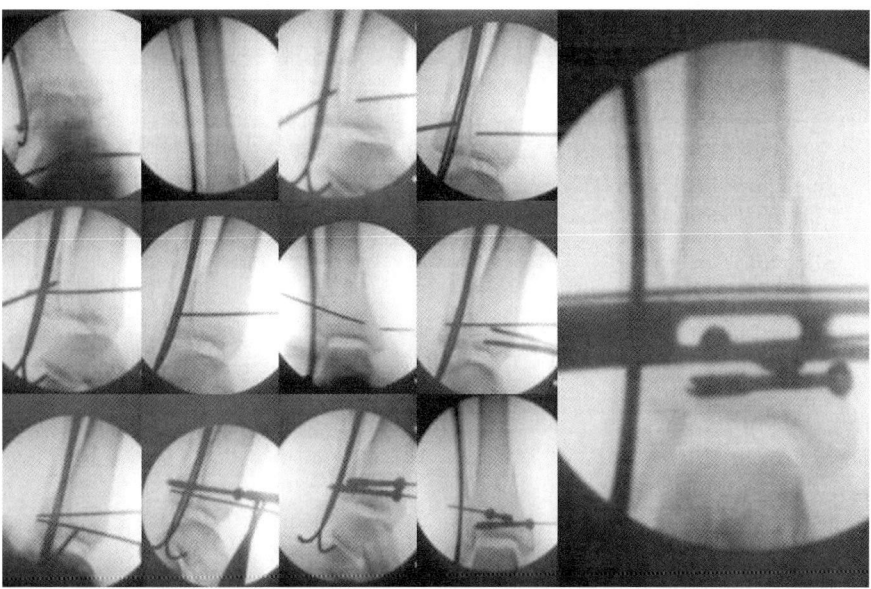

Fig. 5. Successive steps in closed reduction of a pilon fracture with cannulated screws

When the fragment is reduced, one or two guide wires are inserted for internal fixation with cannulated screws.

If closed reduction is impossible, a small antero-medial approach is made for open fixation with small screws.

If opening of the fracture site is required to obtain good reduction, it should be limited and centred over the line of the larger fracture, allowing visualisation of the articular fracture through the fracture window [6].

If opening of the fracture is necessary, consideration is given to a metaphyseal bone graft.

The external hybrid fixator is then assembled. The K-wires that will support the ring are now inserted just above the screws, and positioned around the circumference of the ring in special clamps.

The safe passages must be considered to avoid piercing vital structures. The first wire is inserted from lateral to medial just in front of or behind the fibula. The second wire is inserted from postero-medial to antero-lateral starting just anterior to the neurovascular bundle.

Angulation between the wires of 60° ensures that the fixation is stable. The wires can be positioned on one level as described or at two levels, if space allows, to further increase stability.

After passage through the tissues, the wire is inserted directly into special clamps and locked after being tensioned with special wire-tensioners, usually to 1000-1400 Newtons.

Wires with a central olive are also available. The olive is positioned in contact with the bone to increase stability further or to control free epiphyseal or metaphyseal fragments (Fig. 6). These wires are also locked in special clamps after tensioning. A minimum of three fully tensioned wires is required for good stability.

After wire insertion and tensioning, the ring is attached to a fixator body, which is used as a template for the insertion of two or three screws to the antero-medial face of the tibial diaphysis, after preliminary meta-diaphyseal fracture reduction.

After final reduction, the ring is fixed firmly to the fixator body by tightening the ball joints.

At this point the frame is further stabilised by positioning two reinforcing bars, anteriorly and posteriorly, joining the diaphyseal screws into the ring.

With this frame, which is both stable and flexible, weight-bearing is encouraged in Type A fractures almost immediately, as soon as pain allows, as the fracture does not involve the articular surface.

If the fracture involves the articular surface, load-bearing is forbidden for a period from 8 to 12 weeks, depending on the degree of comminution.

Initial concentration is on active and passive movement of the tibio-tarsal joint to limit stiffness and mould the articular surface (Fig. 7).

From the immediate post-operative period it is essential to apply passive dorsiflexion to the foot, and when resting position a soft bandage from the

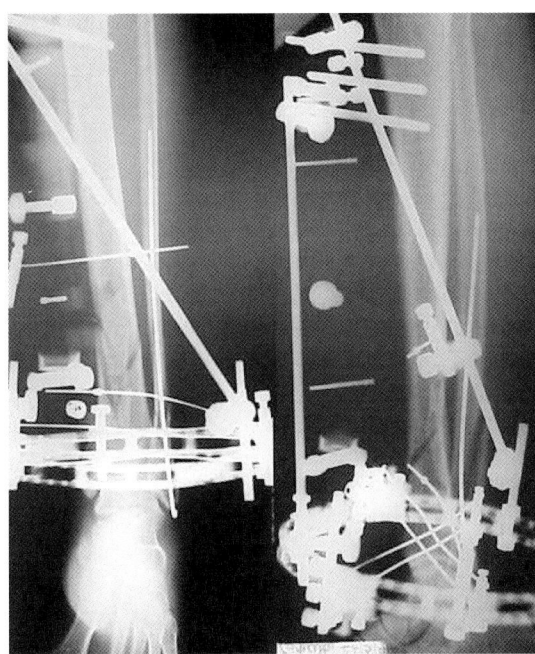

Fig. 6. Extra-articular distal tibial fracture with hybrid implant and opposing wires with olives in the diaphysis to increase stability

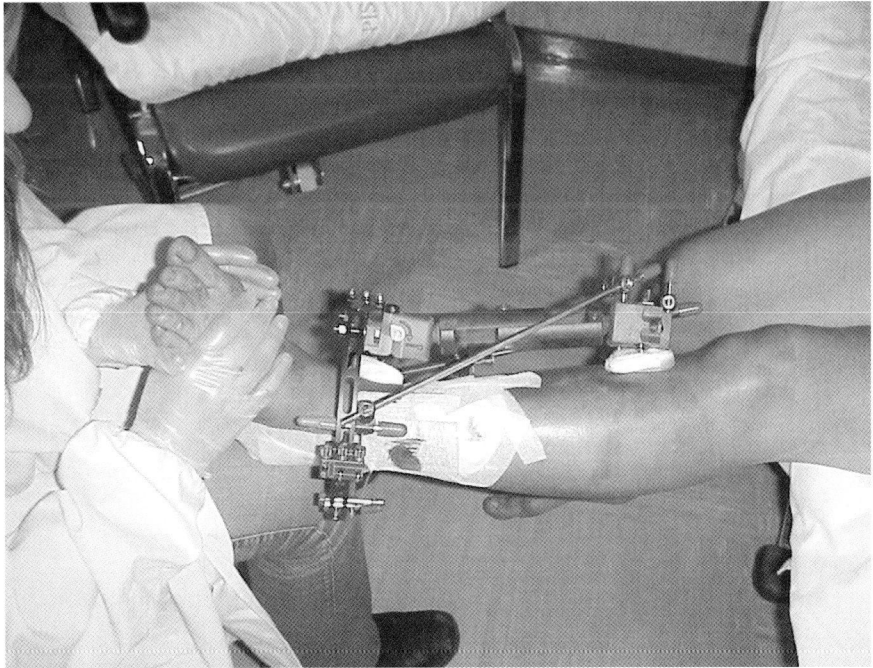

Fig. 7. Physiotherapist performing passive mobilisation to the foot with a hybrid frame in order to reduce stiffness in equinus

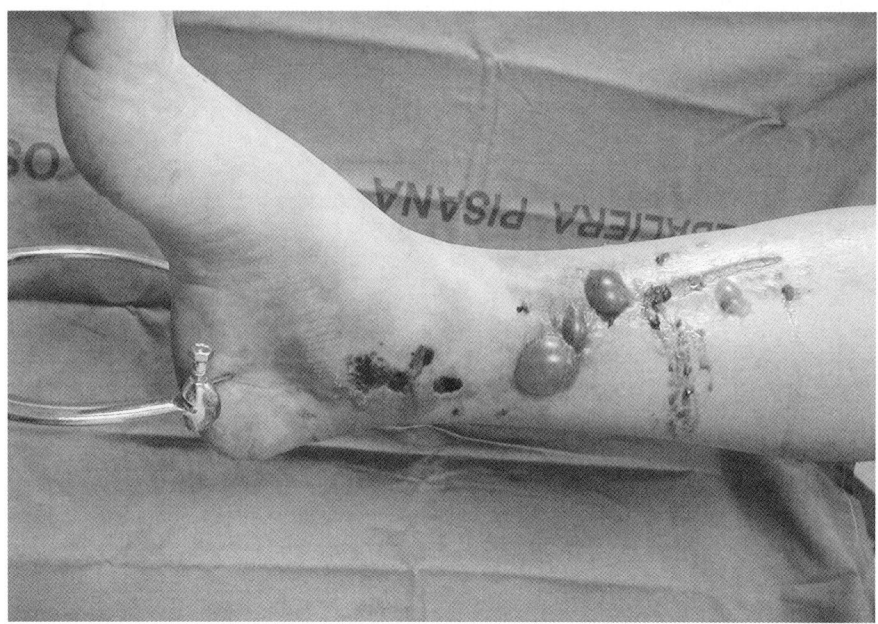

Fig. 8. A limb with blisters of both the serous and haemorrhagic types

fixator to apply passive dorsiflexion. Equinus is a common problem if the fixator is not properly managed and checked.

A hybrid fixator is indicated in Type A distal extra-articular fractures, and Type C1 and C2 fractures, where the articular component is fully reconstructable and the soft tissues not particularly damaged [6].

It is important to check for the presence of blisters, that, particularly if there is haemorrhagic content, indicate underlying soft tissue injury larger than what is immediately visible, and incur a risk of infection six times greater (Fig. 8).

This methodology is not applied in Type B fractures with partial articular involvement and talar subluxation, as the latter is not controlled with this type of fixation.

Application of a hybrid fixator is a challenging procedure and requires familiarity with the use of rings and tensioned wires.

Implant with a Fixator that Bridges the Ankle Without Allowing any Movement

Another possibility for the use of external fixation is application of a bridging fixator as initial stabilisation of a complex fracture of the tibial pilon [2-6].

The fixator places the ankle joint in distraction and temporarily reduces the articular fragments by the mechanism known as ligamentotaxis.

A bridging fixator reduces the need for fibula fixation, as the ligamentotaxis maintains the correct length [11]. An intramedullary K-wire can be used to realign the fibula if required.

The articular fragments of the tibial epiphysis are reduced as already described. The bridging fixator will allow stable joint distraction of about 5 mm, by means of diaphyseal and hindfoot screws parallel with the articular surface in the front plane.

This method has the disadvantage that no movement of the ankle joint is possible.

If the metaphyseal component is particularly comminuted or the hindfoot screws become loose (Fig. 9), it is possible to convert this fixator into a mono-segmental hybrid assembly after 45-60 days with spinal anaesthesia and minimum surgical intervention (Fig. 10).

This permits active and passive mobilisation of the ankle during metaphyseal consolidation, without risk of malunion.

Bridging fixation is indicated in Type B3 fractures with severe articular comminution and in Type C2 and C3 fractures where both articular and metaphyseal comminution is present, with involvement of the soft tissues.

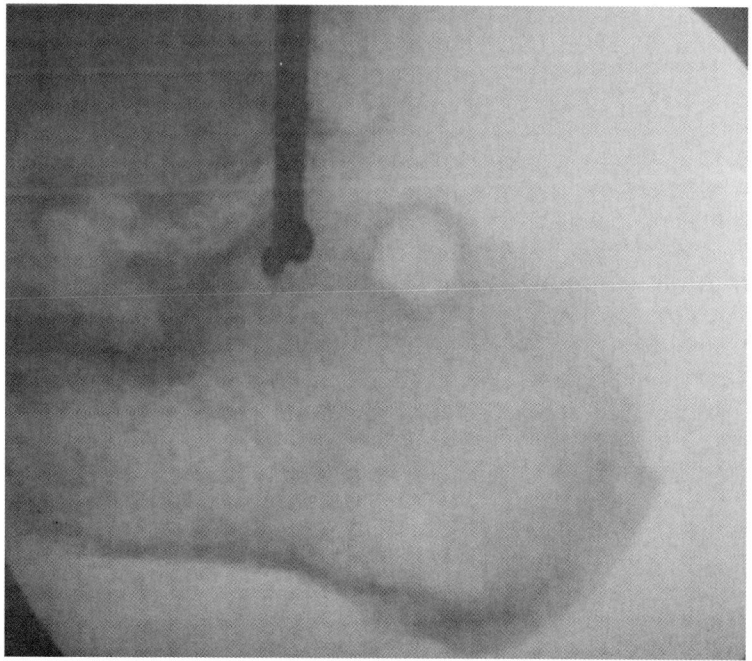

Fig. 9. X-Ray showing the result of previous osteolysis around the calcaneal screw

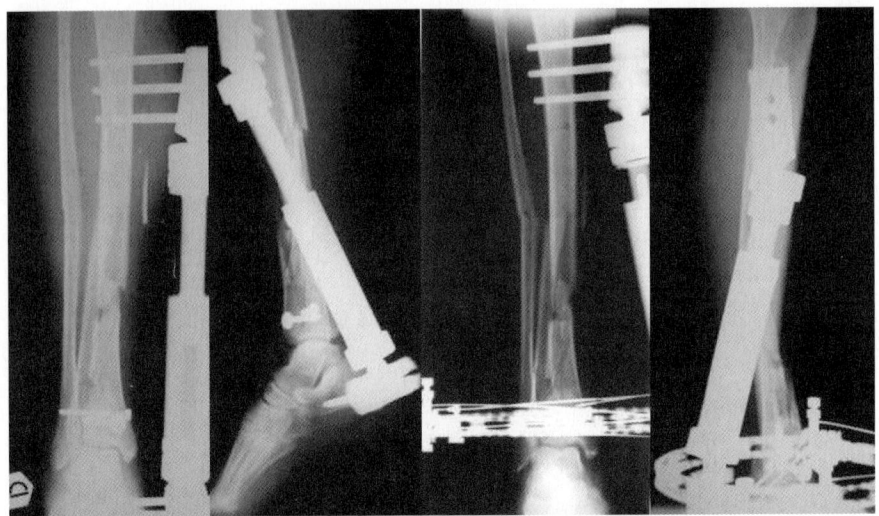

Fig.10. X-Ray of a pilon fracture showing the change from bridging to hybrid assembly

A Bridging Fixator that Allows a Certain Degree of Ankle Movement

The third method involves the use of an articulated external ankle fixator [6, 12], which combines the advantages of a monolateral bridging fixator with early active and passive movement (Fig. 11).

This choice of fixation method has the distinct advantage of limiting joint stiffness and moulding the repaired articular fracture.

Since the centre of rotation of the ankle clamp may not correspond exactly with the centre of rotation of the ankle, slight movement of the fracture is possible during joint movement.

Nevertheless, clinical tests demonstrate that the articulated movement of the ankle does not compromise bone healing [13].

The remarks made previously regarding fibular fixation also apply: the fixator is able to maintain fibula length. Sometimes, however, correct reduction of the fibula may assist in reducing an antero-lateral fragment of the tibial pilon.

On occasions the distal fibula fragment may be incarcerated posteriorly (Fig. 12), in which case ORIF of the fibula is necessary, with a lateral approach and a 1/3 tubular plate.

It is preferable to position the patient in calcaneal traction with the knee flexed 30° so as to permit ligamentotaxis to reduce the articular fragments.

If the soft tissues are compromised, the fixator is positioned without further surgery and left locked.

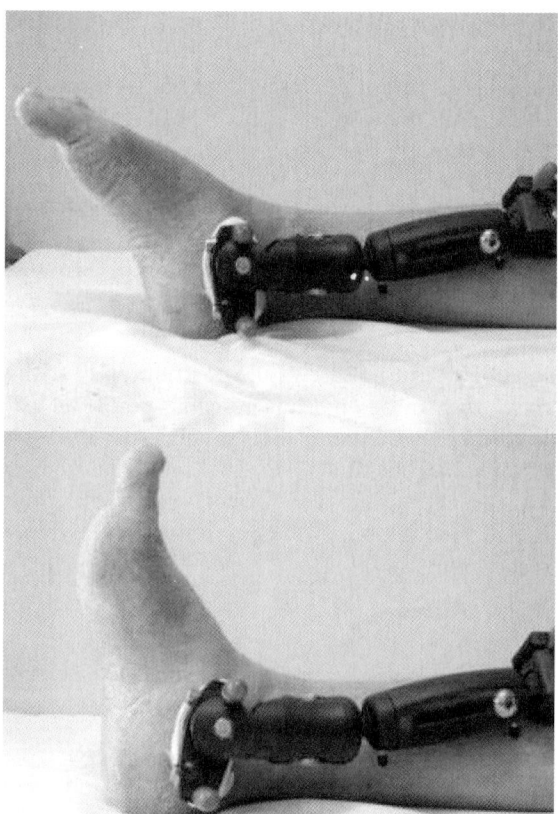

Fig. 11. Clinical image of articulated ankle assembly with joint unlocked and active flexion-extension movements (15°)

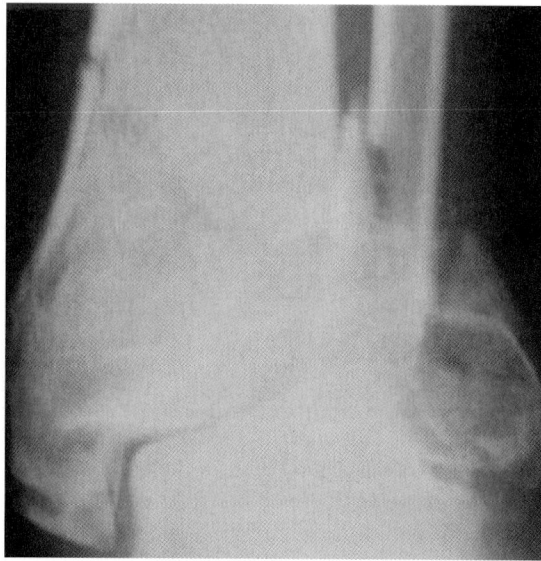

Fig. 12. X-Ray of pilon fracture with incarcerated fibula fragment

When local conditions have improved, reduction and articular fixation can be carried out.

The traction stirrup may disturb the view of the screw insertion point on the medial surface of the calcaneus. To avoid this, the traction wire can be modified into an "S" pattern, shifting the attachment of the stirrup posteriorly to make distal screw insertion easier.

The talar and calcaneal screws are positioned first, using a special template.

A K-wire is inserted into the sinus tarsi, parallel to the talar articular surface, and the template positioned over it.

The metal circle of the template should be in line with the roof of the talus in the lateral view, ensuring that it is over the centre of rotation.

The template is radiolucent, which permits screw hole positioning over the neck of the talus and the calcaneus with sufficient bone tissue around (Fig. 13).

Once the optimum position is reached, the template is steadied in this position by inserting two K-wires, after which the final position is again checked, as it straddles the medial neurovascular bundle. The fixator screws are then inserted parallel to the talar dome in the front plane, using self-drilling screws coated with hydroxyapatite for secure fixation [14].

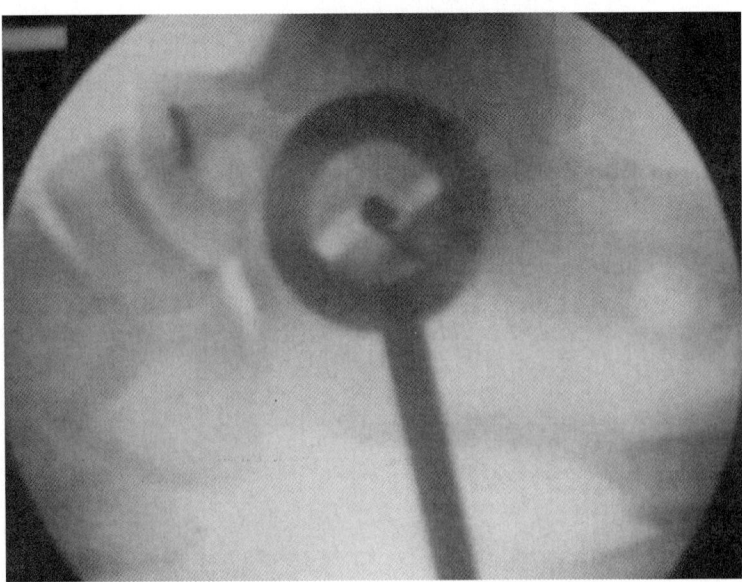

Fig. 13. Image of the guiding template in image intensifier view, showing the screw seats and the centering K-wire

The fixator is applied to the distal screws, and the proximal screws are inserted anteromedially into the tibial diaphysis, using the fixator as template.

The fixator is distracted by about 5 mm to assist joint surface reduction.

At the end of the operation, the distraction is reduced until the joint space has regained a normal appearance.

The ankle clamp is locked with the foot plantigrade.

With the procedure described above, it is often unnecessary to insert a bone graft if closed reduction was successful. It may be necessary for a metaphyseal bone defect, but will be much less frequent compared to the methods that involve wide opening of the fracture. Should a bone graft be required, it should be inserted through a small incision.

The fixator is kept locked in a neutral position. If the conditions of the soft tissues allow, after about one week the ankle clamp is unlocked and assisted movements of the ankle joint are encouraged, up to about 15° of extension and flexion.

It is always necessary to position a bandage to prevent forefoot equinus.

If the hindfoot also tends to equinus, after having performed active or passive articulation exercises it is preferable to re-tighten the ankle clamp with the foot plantigrade. Gradual weight-bearing can be allowed, starting from the first few days, according to the state of the soft tissues.

Use of an intermittent foot-pump for reducing the oedema and aiding venous return may be beneficial.

Use of the foot-pump is also highly important in the stages preceding the operation, particularly when this period becomes extended due to adverse local or general conditions.

If the metaphyseal component is particularly compromised, weight-bearing is postponed up to 45-60 days. When partial weight-bearing is considered desirable, dynamization is recommended.

The fixator is removed when well-formed callus is seen on X-Ray.

It is good practice to remove the fixator but leave the screws *in situ* and permit full weight-bearing for 7-10 days if there is any doubt of the quality of the metaphyseal consolidation. After this period, the screws can be removed if the patient does not feel pain and if there are no radiographic changes.

The bridging fixator with the possibility of articular movement is used in Type B fractures and particularly in Type C2 and C3 fractures with significant soft tissue damage, which will inevitably sustain a high incidence of complications if treated by ORIF with a plate.

If the external bridging fixator is used for initial fixation in the presence of a severe open wound or other massive involvement of the soft tissues, examination of the fracture can be completed with CT. This is much more usefully performed after fixator application with some distraction.

A CT performed urgently when the talus is wedged in the tibial mortar results in overlapping images that are poor for the purposes of pre-operative planning.

In the case of a high degree of metaphyseal comminution area or if the hind-foot screws become loose, the articulating implant can also be converted into a monosegmental hybrid implant with tensioned wires on a ring.

Treatment Algorithm

Open Fractures, of any AO Classification

A bridging articulated fixator is applied as an emergency (Fig. 14), with the clamp locked in a neutral position. Wound debridement, lavage, subsequent soft tissue management and plastic closure of any defect are carried out as advised by the plastic surgeon.

The fixation of the articular surface must be as minimally invasive as possible, with wires and small diameter cannulated screws (Fig. 15).

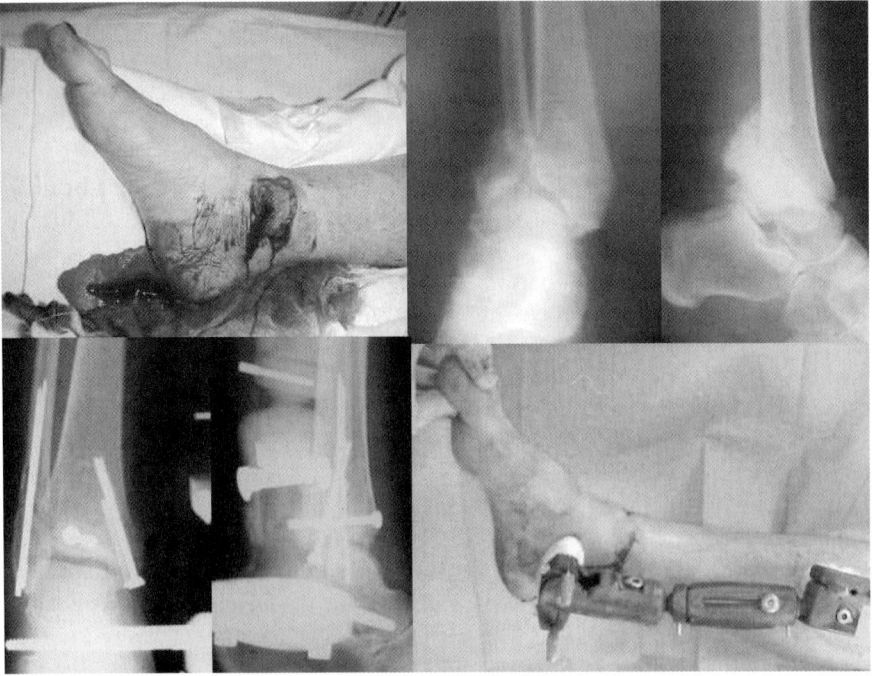

Fig. 14. Treatment of an open tibial pilon fracture with an articulated bridging fixator, which was in this case radiolucent

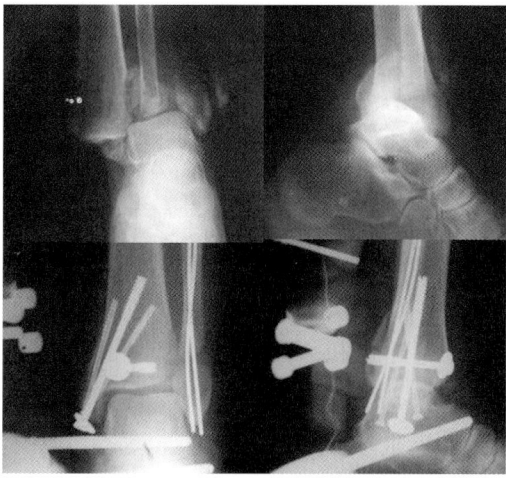

Fig. 15. X-Ray with fixation of an open fracture with wires and cannulated screws

Type A Fractures

A hybrid fixator is used with a ring and tensioned wires, stabilisation bars and early weight-bearing.

During the stage of callus maturation, the implant is made less rigid by removal of the bars (Fig. 16).

The intrinsic elasticity of the tensioned wires makes fixator dynamization unnecessary.

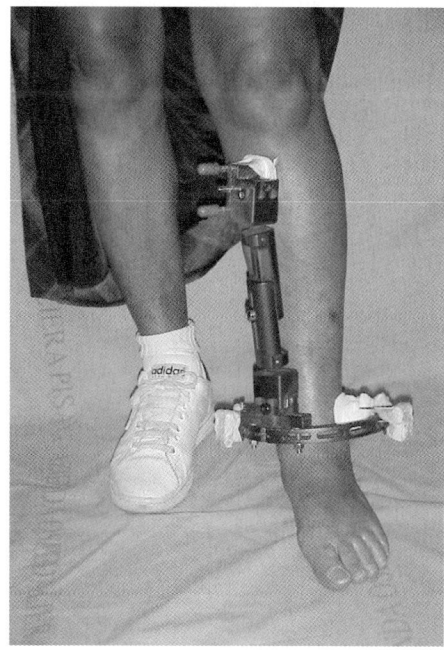

Fig. 16. Clinical image of hybrid implant following removal of the tensioning bars to reduce fixator rigidity

Type C1 and C2 Fractures

If these fractures have articular fragments that are sufficiently large and soft tissues that are not particularly compromised, the articular surface is reconstructed (Fig. 17) following restoration of fibula length. A hybrid fixator is applied with wires positioned just above the screws that secure the articular fragments.

Weight-bearing must be forbidden for at least two months.

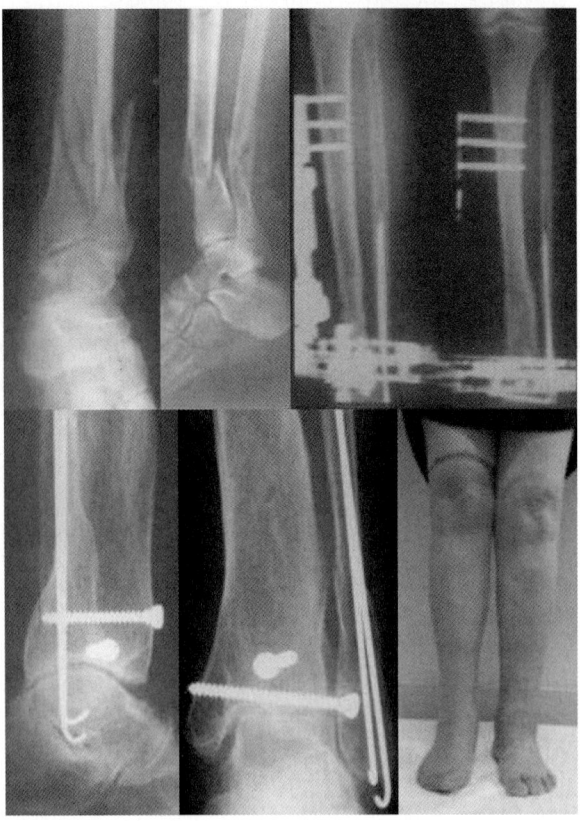

Fig. 17. A Type C2 pilon fracture: reduction and fixation with screws and hybrid fixator

Type C2 and C3 Fractures

These usually present significant articular comminution and serious soft tissue involvement, frequently with associated haemorrhagic blisters (Fig. 18).

An articulated bridging fixator is applied; fixation of the articular surface may be concurrent or deferred, depending on the condition of the soft tissues.

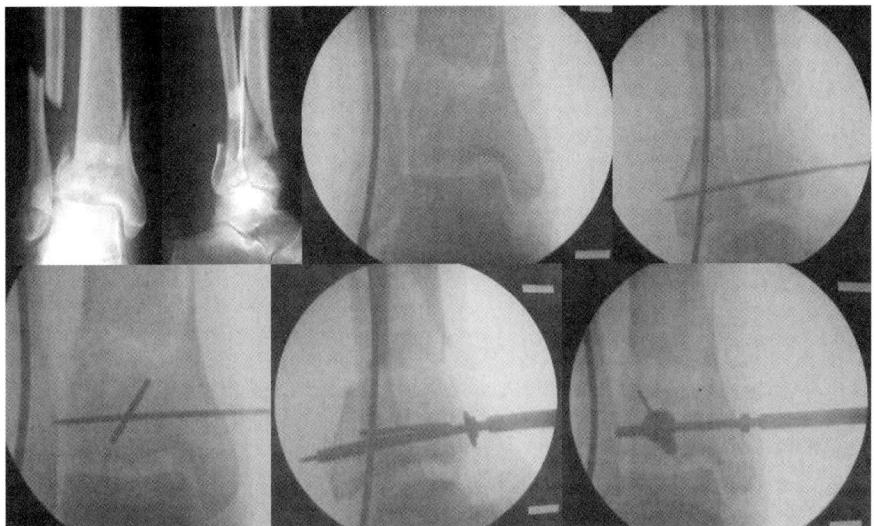

Fig. 18. Illustration of reduction a Type C3 fracture with a bridging fixator

Conclusions

According to the data in the recent literature, the treatment method described here has strongly reduced short-term complications such as deep infection, amputation and non union [15].

However, usage of this method does not seem to have had a positive impact on long-term complications, which are mainly related to post-traumatic arthrosis.

It permits rapid healing of the soft tissue, including any procedure carried out by the plastic surgeon.

It allows the period of hospitalisation to be reduced and the patient to become independent more rapidly.

It is a method that allows biological healing without additionally compromising the soft tissues, preventing extensive surgical exposure.

Lastly, this method does not require further surgery to remove metal implants, except for cannulated screws that are easily removed with minimum incisions.

It is a relatively simple method that nevertheless requires a good support system, good pre-operative planning and continuous monitoring of the patients until full healing has occurred.

References

1. Ruedi TP, Algower M (1979) The operative treatment of intra-articular fractures of the lower end of the tibia. Clin Orthop 138:105-110

2. Bone L, Stegemann P, McNamara K et al (1993) External fixation of severely comminuted and open tibial pilon fractures. Clin Orthop 292:101-107
3. Tornetta P III, Weiner L, Bergman M et al (1993) Pilon fractures: treatment with combined internal and external fixation. J Orthop Trauma 7:489-496
4. Saleh M, Shanahan MDG, Fern ED (1993) Intra-articular fractures of the distal tibia: surgical management by limited internal fixation and articulated distraction. Injury 24:37-40
5. Marsh JL, Bonar S, Nepola JV et al (1995) Use of an articuled external fixator for fractures of the tibial plafond. J Bone Joint Surg Am 77:1498-1509
6. Bonar SK, Marsh JL (1994) Tibial plafond fractures, changing principles of treatment. J Am Acad Orthop Surg 2:297-305
7. Müller ME, Nazarian S, Koch P et al (1990) The comprensive classification of fractures of long bone. Springer, Berlin Heidelberg New York, pp 170-179
8. Thordarson DB (2000) Complicanze dopo il trattamento delle fratture del pilone tibiale: strategie per la prevenzione e la cura. J Am Acad Orthop Surg 8:253-265
9. Murphy CP, D'Ambrosia R, Dabezies EJ (1994) The small pin circular fixator for distal tibial pilon fractures with soft tissue compromise. Orthopedics 14:283-290
10. Manca M, Marchetti S, Faldini C, Faldini A (2002) Combined percutaneous internal fixation and external fixation treatment of type C tibial plafond fractures: a review of 22 cases. Scientific Exhibit N° SE50, Proceedings of the 69th American Academy of Orthopaedics Surgeon, Vol 3, p 749
11. Mast JW, Spiegel PG, Pappas JN (1998) Fractures of the tibial pilon. Clin Orthop Rel Res 230:68-81
12. Lavini F, Renzi Brivio L, Leso P (1987) Il trattamento con fissatori esterni nelle fratture articolari di ginocchio e tibio tarsica. SERTOT Proceedings 29(2):249-252
13. Bonar SK, Marsh JL (1993) Unilateral external fixation for severe pilon fractures. Foot Ankle 7:489-496
14. Magyar G, Toksvig-Larsen S, Moroni A (1997) Hydroxyapatite coating of threaded pins enhances fixation. J Bone Joint Surg Br 79:487-489
15. McFerran MA, Smith SW, Boulas HJ, Schwartz HS (1992) Complications encountered in the treatment of pilon fractures. J Orthop Trauma 6:195-200

Open Fractures

Criteria for Treating Open Fractures

E.J. Müller, G. Muhr

Introduction

The incidence of severe lower leg trauma seems to be increasing in high-level trauma centres. This is probably due to the widespread use of automobile crash protection systems that mainly protect the upper body and head, but leave the lower part of the legs unprotected.

The treatment of severe tibial pilon fractures remains a difficult problem for many orthopaedic trauma surgeons, because the features of the injury, which include metaphyseal comminution, damage to the articular surface and poor soft tissue coverage, result in a high incidence of complications and unsatisfactory results [1-10] (Fig. 1). These include a high incidence of infection, arthrodesis of the tibiotarsal joint and amputation [11], whereas the low-energy pilon fracture, which can be reconstructed anatomically with an internal fixation system, has quite a good prognosis.

Since the classic articles by Ruedi, Matter and Allgower were published in 1968 and 1969 [12, 13], the outcomes of low-energy pilon fractures have markedly improved owing to the development of an algorithm for standardised treatment that considers anatomic reconstruction of the surface of the joint and proper management of the soft tissue as the most important factors in obtaining a good result. The basic steps in treatment are reconstruction of fibula length and stabilisation to help reduce the metaphyseal fragments, anatomical reconstruction of the joint surface, support for the medial tibial column and bone graft at the level of the most proximal fracture line, if necessary.

It was therefore possible to improve the functional result by open reduction and stable internal fixation, but when high-energy fractures were treated with the same method, significant complications resulted. Reported rates of deep infection varied between 6% and 55%, and soft tissue complications were

Chirurgische Klinik und Poliklinik, BG-Kliniken Bergmannsheil, Ruhruniversität Bochum

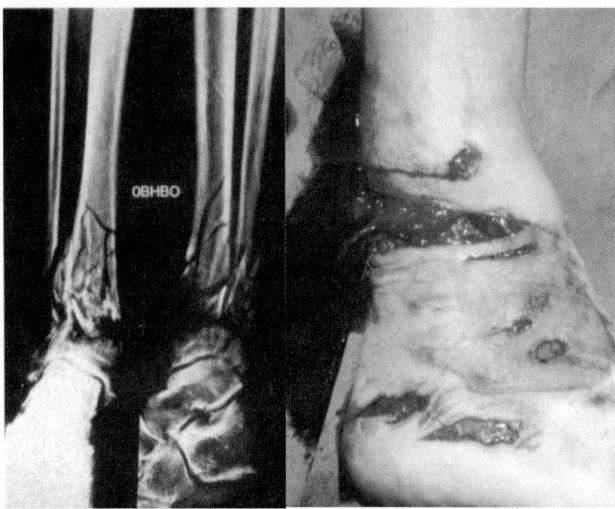

Fig. 1. Initial X-Rays and clinical appearance

between 11% and 27% [11, 14-17]. These different results demonstrated that not all pilon fractures were the same, with results strictly correlated to the type of fracture. High-energy impact fractures, with comminution and soft tissue damage, present a poorer prognosis than those resulting from low-energy torsion, independent of the method of treatment [6-8, 11]. The results reflect the impact of the complications, particularly infection or wound healing [3, 10]. It follows that the treatment protocol for high-energy fractures with serious soft tissue injury requires modification. Proper reconstruction of the joint surface must be achieved without causing further damage to the soft tissues. To improve results, staged protocols are required, with limited internal fixation and external fixation, or initial external fixation and delayed open reduction and internal fixation, or application of a hybrid external fixation system. The use of these protocols can significantly reduce the frequency of complications [3, 5, 8, 9, 18-23].

Despite this, each method has its limitations, and the functional result for severe open fractures is still poor, so that these patients are left with residual psychosocial disability. Because of this some authors have proposed that these patients might benefit more from early amputation than reconstruction, which requires major commitments of time and economic resources.

Soft Tissue Anatomy

The soft tissue coverage around the tibiotarsal joint is rather thin. The skin receives its blood supply from the deep fascia via perforating vessels from the dorsal arteries of the foot, and the posterior tibial and peroneal arteries. The superficial venous system comprises the internal saphenous vein that travels with the saphenous nerve in front of the medial malleolus and along the medial surface of the tibia towards the knee, and the external saphenous vein, which runs with the sural nerve behind the lateral malleolus and up the centre of the calf. Destruction of the veins during the injury or operation may cause the complications of venous stasis and recurrent swelling of the foot.

Following a high-energy tibial pilon fracture, compartment syndrome may develop due to the strong coverage of the four different compartments by the deep fascia. The anterior compartment contains the tibialis anterior muscle, extensor hallucis longus, extensor digitorum, peroneus tertius and the anterior tibial vein, artery and nerve. At the level of the tibiotarsal joint, these structures pass deep to the superior extensor retinaculum, with the neurovascular bundle lying between the tendons of extensor digitorum longus and extensor hallucis longus. The lateral compartment contains the peroneus brevis and peroneus longus and the lateral popliteal nerve, which pierces the deep fascia to become the superficial peroneal nerve at the junction of the middle and distal thirds of the leg, dividing in a variable pattern into two branches superficial to the superior retinaculum. The posterior superficial compartment contains the gastrocnemius, soleus and plantaris muscles. The deep posterior compartment contains flexor digitorum longus, the tibialis posterior and flexor hallucis longus, and the posterior tibial neurovascular bundle. The latter contributes to the vascular anastomosis around the ankle joint, and passes under the flexor retinaculum, behind the medial malleolus with the flexor tendons.

Classification

The complete AO fracture classification with the three main groups of A, B and C [24] has been generally accepted, despite the documented inter- and intra-observer variability within the system [25-27]. It has been modified by the OTA.

In open fractures, the soft tissue wound is classified according to Gustilo and Anderson [28].

The attempt made by Collins and Temple [29] to draw up a prognostic classification of open wounds may be useful for decision-making. In their description, pilon compression fractures were considered Types IIIB or IV open fractures. In their series, 60% of the Type IV wounds became infected, and of these 33% required amputation.

In complicated cases with chronic infection, Weiland and colleagues' classification may be useful for decision-making [30].

Treatment Protocol

Whereas initial reconstruction and internal fixation may still be applied with good results in low-energy closed fractures with minimum soft tissue trauma, as was suggested in the early era of operative treatment, the protocol has changed over the last ten years for high-energy wounds. Because of the high frequency of complications, which mainly consist of secondary infection due to the destruction of soft tissue coverage, many authors have proposed a staged protocol with initial external fixation, using a standard external fixator, a hybrid fixator or even a fixator with hinges, with or without limited percutaneous stabilisation, followed by delayed internal fixation. Using this protocol, numerous publications have reported a significant reduction of infection, especially in complex fractures with severe soft tissue damage [5, 7, 14, 18, 20, 31-34].

There is little information regarding the management of open pilon fractures. Ovadia and Beals [11] reported 25 second and third degree open pilon fractures, 9 of which became infected. In open fractures with significant soft tissue loss, their protocol followed the same principles that had been established for treating open long bone fractures, using external fixation, repeated and scheduled wound debridement, soft tissue coverage and final stabilisation of the fracture [35-39]. However, modification of the protocol became necessary, since the involved joint is weight-bearing and has poor soft tissue coverage. Generally, the method chosen for initial stabilisation of open tibial pilon fractures is application of an external fixation device (Fig. 2). Whenever possible, we recommend initial reconstruction of the articular surface through small incisions using K-wires and/or small fragment screws. If initial reduction is not perfect, as is likely in Type C injuries, final reconstruction of the articular surface is simpler if the main fragments have already been approximated. This also reduces pressure on the soft tissues.

Due to the damaging effects of immobilizing the tibiotarsal and subtalar joints, use of a hybrid external fixator is recommended, in which epiphyseal purchase is achieved with a ring and tensioned wires, and attached to the diaphysis with unilateral half-pins [1, 4, 9, 22, 23]. It stabilises the main articular surface without bridging the ankle joint, and use of thin wires may cause fewer soft tissue problems compared to the use of large pins. The first papers regarding this technique were rather promising, although serious complications were also reported, due to infection of the wire tracks with consequent osteomyelitis [4, 9, 10, 22]. However, an external bridging fixator is recommended in severe open fractures with soft tissue damage because the bone screws can be positioned far away from the damaged soft tissues, thus preventing local complications.

A useful principle of treating open fractures is to shorten the fracture site by 2-3 cm, instead of the initial reconstruction of fibula length. This lowers the tension in the surrounding soft tissues, and increases local perfusion. Indeed this can help soft tissue recovery and even facilitate initial wound suture in Type I open fractures. Once soft tissue coverage is complete, partial restoration of length can be made if the original shortening was greater than 2 cm, by means of distraction with an external fixator (Figs. 3-5). Otherwise final osteosynthesis is performed in the shortened position.

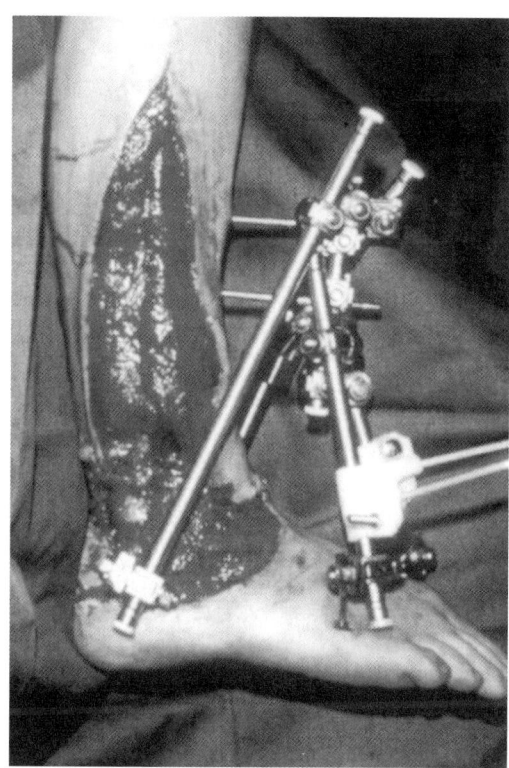

Fig. 2. Primary external fixation with a bridging fixator, shortening to release soft tissue tension, debridement and reconstruction of the vascular injury

If articular reconstruction is possible with minimal exposure, the external fixator can be used as a final stabilisation method until the fracture is healed. However, particularly in fractures with extended metaphyseal comminution, this method results in a longer healing time and a higher frequency of non-union or malunion compared to ORIF with a plate. Also, the incidence of pin track infection and resulting sequelae must be considered [3, 8-10].

Instead of open plate fixation the metaphyseal fracture can be stabilised with a minimally invasive plate osteosynthesis. In this technique a precontoured plate - preferably a plate which allows screw insertion with angular stability - is placed over the antero-medial aspect of the distal tibia through a small incision over the medial malleolus, with the screws inserted through stab incisions. This minimises the trauma to the surrounding soft tissues. If the medial aspect of the distal tibia is exposed due to loss of soft tissue envelope, plating can be performed immediately before covering the defect with a free vascularised flap. In crush injuries with severe comminution of the joint area primary arthrodesis should be considered to salvage the limb [35]. However, in the presence of significant bone loss, this may become exceptionally difficult [35, 40, 41].

Complete wound coverage is usually obtained with either a variable thickness skin graft or a regional flap following sequential debridement in Types I and II open wounds.

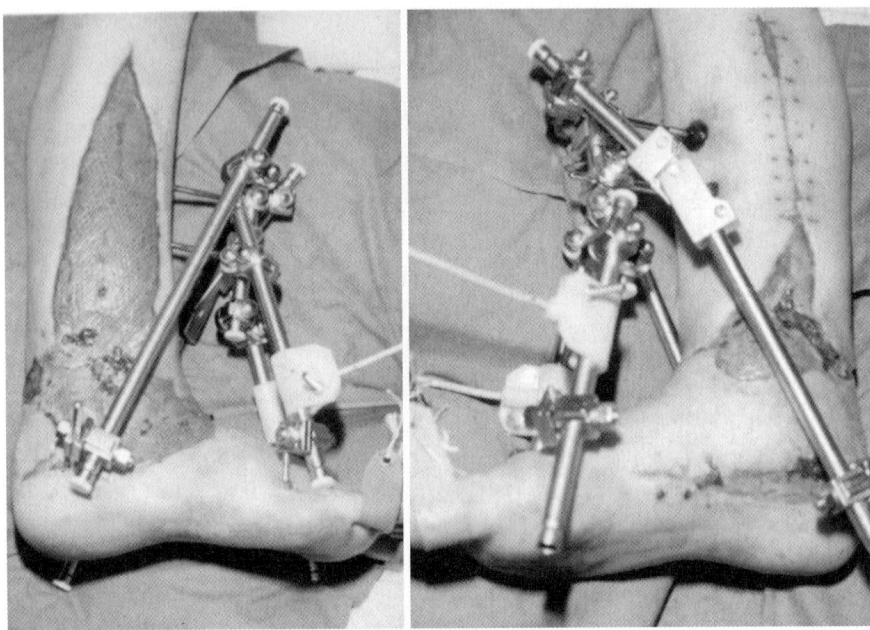

Fig. 3. Restoration of soft tissue coverage with variable thickness skin graft

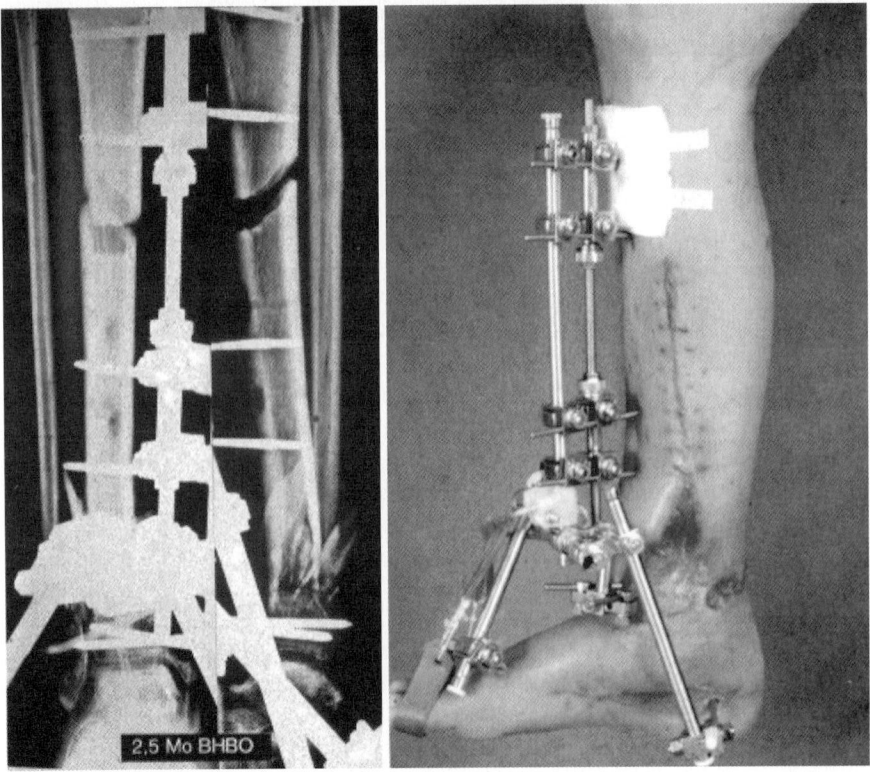

Fig. 4. Bone reconstruction with transport of the proximal tibial segment into the bone defect

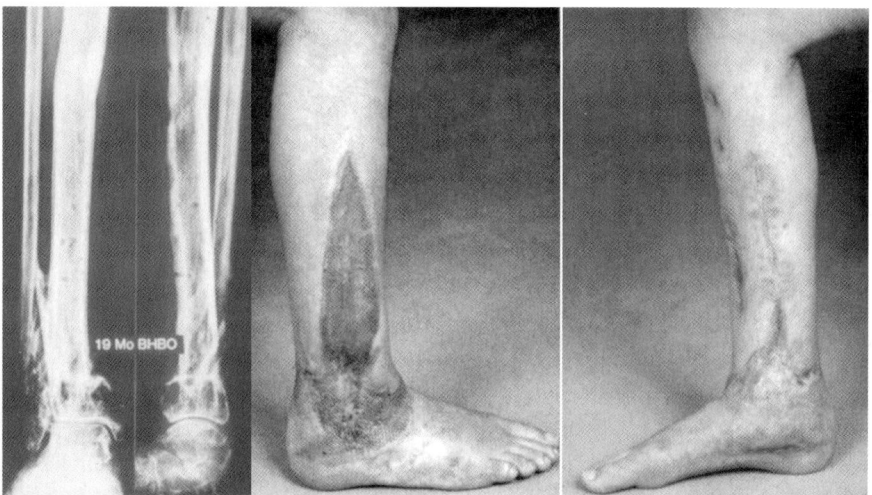

Fig. 5. Final clinical and X-Ray results after 19 months of treatment. The patient is able to fully weight-bear; the ROM of the tibiotarsal and subtalar joints is significantly reduced

It may be necessary to cover the defect in Type III open fractures with a free vascularized muscle flap [30, 36-39]. Precise planning of the soft tissue coverage should involve a plastic surgeon from the beginning, to avoid unnecessary repetitive debridements. It is essential to achieve complete coverage as soon as possible, depending on the local and general condition of the patient.

Salvage or Amputation?

In choosing between salvage and amputation, six parameters require consideration: expected final function, aesthetic appearance and presence of chronic swelling, pain or lack of sensation, time required for completion of treatment, cost of the treatment and psychological factors. Also the premorbid condition of the lower leg and the contralateral extremity should be evaluated [42].

Stabilisation of a fracture is generally not the biggest problem. The degree of comminution serves as an indicator of the amount of energy absorbed. In comparable cases, severely comminuted or complex open fractures have less chance of functional recovery than single or complex closed fractures. Sanders and colleagues have demonstrated that, despite excellent reconstruction, the result is poor in patients with severe open fractures at the ankle and talus, and early below knee amputation would have been preferable [35]. Other authors have reported similar results [40, 43].

Division of the posterior tibial nerve generally tips the balance in favour of amputation, when associated with severe bone or soft tissue injury. Damage to the nerve produces an anaesthetic foot, secondary deformity from denervation of the intrinsic muscles, and possible neuropathic pain. The foot may have moderate functionality, but the lack of sensation will cause additional complications, as in patients with diabetic neuropathy.

Division of the posterior tibial artery is a relative contraindication to functional salvage, unless the section is clean. Soft tissue coverage in the distal third of the leg, necessary for adequate vascular and neural repair, is poor. Damage to the venous and lymphatic systems may lead to serious chronic swelling, markedly compromising healing and functionality.

Amputation should be performed above the injured area and the stump covered with skin without scars and with normal sensation. The amputation level should also allow for optimum adaptation to a well functioning prosthesis with a good aesthetic appearance. In the open pilon fracture it is possible to perform an amputation below the knee with a stump long enough for optimum adaptation to a prosthesis.

Salvage may be satisfactory in selected patients, but in some patients with other significant local problems with soft tissues or bone, or in patients compromised systemically due to diabetes, malnutrition, smoking or immunodeficiency, early amputation may be a better option [40, 42].

Summary

A staged protocol with an initial external fixation system associated with minimally invasive reconstruction of the articular surface and delayed internal fixation is recommended in open tibial pilon fractures. Treatment of the soft tissues is performed as for open long bone fractures, with repeated debridement and early coverage, with a free flap if necessary. In cases of severe articular comminution, the option of arthrodesis of the tibiotarsal joint should be considered. In many cases, it is possible to salvage the lower extremity in Type C open lesions, but this is associated with a high incidence of permanent disability. In these cases, delayed amputation in severe open and complex fractures may be the preferred method.

References

1. Barbierei R, Schenk R, Koval K et al (1996) Hybrid external fixation in the treatment of tibial plafond fractures. Clin Orthop 332:16-22
2. Bonar SK, Marsh JL (1993) Unilateral external fixation for severe pilon fractures. Foot Ankle 14:57-64
3. Bone LB, Stegemann B, McNamara K, Seibel R (1993) External fixation of severely comminuted and open tibial pilon fractures. Clin Orthop 292:101-107
4. Griffiths GP, Thordarson DB (1996) Tibial plafond fractures: limited internal fixation and a hybrid external fixator. Foot Ankle Int 17:444-448
5. Höntzsch D, Karnatz N, Jansen T (1990) Ein- und zweizeitige Versorgung der schweren Pilon-tibiale-Fraktur. Aktuelle Traumatol 20:199-204

6.   Marsh JL, Rattay RE, Dulaney T (1997) Results of ankle arthrodesis for treatment of supramalleolar non-union and ankle arthrosis. Foot Ankle Int 18:138-143
7.   Muhr G, Breitfuß H (1993) Complication after pilon fracture. In: Tscherne H, Schatzker J (eds) Major fractures of the pilon, the talus and the calcaneus. Springer, Berlin Heidelberg New York, p 65
8.   Rommens PM, Claes P, De Boodt P et al (1994) Therapeutisches Vorgehen und Langzeitergebnisse bei der Pilonfraktur in Abhängigkeit vom primären Weichteilschaden. Unfallchirurg 97:39-46
9.   Tornetta P III, Weiner L, Bergmann M et al (1993) Pilon fractures: treatment with combined internal and external fixation. J Orthop Trauma 7:489-496
10. Wyrsch B, McFerran MA, McAndrew M et al (1996) Operative treatment of fractures of the tibial plafond: a randomised prospective study. J Bone Joint Surg Am 78:1646-1657
11. Ovadia DN, Beals RK (1986) Fractures of the tibial plafond. J Bone Joint Surg Am 68:543-551
12. Ruedi T, Matter P, Allgower M (1968) Die intra-artikulären Frakturen des distalen Unterschenkelendes. Helv Chir Acta 35:556-582
13. Ruedi T, Allgower M (1969) Fractures of the lower end of the tibia into the ankle joint. Injury 1:92-99
14. Borelli J Jr, Ellis E (2002) Pilon fractures: assessment and treatment. Orthop Clin North Am 33:231-245
15. Dillin L, Slabaugh P (1986) Delayed wound healing, infection, and non-union following open reduction and internal fixation of tibial plafond fractures. J Trauma 26:1119-1119
16. McFerran MA, Smith SW, Boulas HJ, Schartz HS (1992) Complications encountered in the treatment of pilon fractures. J Orthop Trauma 6:195-200
17. Pierce R, Heinrich J (1979) Comminuted intra-articular fractures of the distal tibia. J Trauma 19:828-832
18. Sirkin M, Sanders R, DiPasquale T, Herscovici D Jr (1999) A staged protocol for soft tissue management in the treatment of complex pilon fractures. J Orthop Trauma 13:78-84
19. Kilian O, Bündner MS, Horas U et al (2002) Langzeitergebnisse nach operativer Versorgung von Pilon-tibial-Frakturen. Chirurg 73:65-72
20. Patterson MJ, Cole JD (1999) Two-staged delayed open reduction and internal fixation of severe pilon fractures. J Orthop Trauma 13:85-91
21. Watson JT, Moed BR, Karges DE, Cramer KE (2000) Pilon fractures. Treatment protocol based on the severity of soft tissue injury. Clin Orthop 375:78-90
22. Anglen JO (1999) Early outcome of hybrid external fixation for fracture of the distal tibia. J Orthop Trauma 13:92-97
23. Beals TC (2001) Application of ring fixators in complex foot and ankle trauma. Orthop Clin North Am 32:205-214
24. Muller ME, Allgower M, Schneider R, Willenegger H (1991) Manual of internal fixation: techniques recommended by the AO/ASIF group, 3rd edn. Springer, Berlin Heidelberg New York
25. Dirschl DR, Adams GL (1997) A critical assessment of factors influencing reliability in the classification of fractures, using the tibial plafond as a model. J Orthop Trauma 11:471-476
26. Martin JS, Marsh JL, Bonar SK et al (1997) Assessment of the AO/ASIF fracture classification for the distal tibia. J Orthop Trauma 11:477-483

27. Swiontkowski MF, Sands AK, Agel J et al (1997) Interobserver variation in the AO/OTA fracture classification system for pilon fractures. Is there a problem? J Orthop Trauma 11:467-470

28. Gustilo RB, Anderson JT (1976) Prevention of infection in the treatment of one thousand and twenty-five open fractures of long bones: retrospective and prospective analyses. J Bone Joint Surg Am 58:453-458

29. Collins DN, Temple SD (1989) Open joint injuries. Clin Orthop 178:54-63

30. Weiland AJ, Moore JR, Daniel RK (1984) The efficacy of free tissue transfer in the treatment of osteomyelitis. J Bone Joint Surg Am 66:181-193

31. Bastian L, Blauth M, Thermann H, Tscherne H (1995) Verschiedene therapiekonzepte bei schweren Frakturen des pilon tibiale (Typ-C-verletzungen). Unfallchirurg 98:551-558

32. Scheck M (1965) Treatment of comminuted distal tibial fractures by combined dual-pin fixation and limited open reduction. J Bone Joint Surg Am 47:1537-1553

33. Pugh KJ, Wolinsky PR, McAndrew MP, Johnson KD (1999) Tibial pilon fractures: a comparison of treatment methods. J Trauma 47:937-941

34. Thordarson DB (2000) Complications after treatment of tibial pilon fractures: prevention and management strategies. J Am Acad Orthop Surg 8:253-265

35. Sanders R, Pappas J, Mast J, Helfet D (1992) The salvage of open grade IIIB ankle and talus fractures. J Orthop Trauma 6:201-208

36. Caudle RJ, Stern PJ (1987) Severe open fractures of the tibia. J Bone Joint Surg Am 69:801-807

37. Cierny G III, Byrd HS, Jones RE (1983) Primary versus delayed soft tissue coverage for severe open tibial fractures. Clin Orthop 178:54-63

38. Hanson ST (1987) The type IIIC tibial fracture. J Bone Joint Surg Am 69:799-780

39. Yaremchuck MJ, Brumback RJ, Manson PN et al (1987) Acute and definitive management of traumatic osteocutaneous defects of the lower extremity. Plast Reconstr Surg 80:1-12

40. Cierny G III, Cook WG, Mader JT (1989) Ankle arthrodesis in the presence of ongoing sepsis: indications, methods and results. Orthop Clin North Am 20:709-721

41. Morrey BF, Weidemenn GP (1980) Complications and long term results of ankle arthrodesis following trauma. J Bone Joint Surg Am 62:777-784

42. Hanson ST (2001) Salvage or amputation after complex foot and ankle trauma. Orthop Clin North Am 32:181-186

43. Marsh JL, Bonar SK, Nepola JV et al (1995) Use of an articulated external fixator for fractures of the tibial plafond. J Bone Joint Surg Am 77:1498-1509

Soft Tissue Reconstruction of Complex Wounds

L. VAIENTI

Because of the complex nature of tibial pilon fractures, and the difficulties that are presented during reconstruction, a wide variety of treatment methods has been proposed by different authors [1-8].

For years there was no satisfactory solution, but in recent decades sophisticated, innovative techniques have been developed to restore the soft issues, often as a single stage procedure. This allows the surgeon to undertake increasingly complex skeletal reconstruction programmes. Every repair made on the deep structures, whether bony, tendinous or neurovascular, is destined to failure if there is no good quality soft tissue coverage.

The latter should therefore be the first objective of a surgical approach, which aims initially at minimizing the risk of a contaminated wound becoming septic.

If the skin integrity is broken by violent trauma and there is direct contamination with micro-organisms, an ischaemic and hypoxic area is created that favours the virulence of anaerobic bacteria otherwise checked by normal oxygen levels.

Also, the nature of the contamination caused by the penetration of sand or dirt inside the wound will foster the development of infection. The lower limb is more susceptible to infection because of the relative ischaemia caused by the smaller number of capillaries present in the skin of the lower limbs and the low capacity of the neutrophil leukocytes to migrate to the infected area.

Finally, the presence of tissue dead spaces as a result of loss of substance or

Unità di Chirurgia Plastica Ricostruttiva degli Arti, Istituto di Chirurgia Plastica Ricostruttiva, Università degli Studi di Milano, Istituto Policlinico San Donato

Reconstruction of the Distal Third of the Leg with Regional Island Flaps

These are ideal reconstruction solutions in trauma of the tibial pilon, since they originate remotely from the periphery of the wound and have reliable neurovascular pedicles.

Sural Flap

The sural flap is a reliable flap with a long, continuous pedicle. It is a fasciocutaneous island flap and is currently the most widely used for reconstruction of the distal third of the leg (Fig. 1). It is taken from the posterior surface of the leg with a distal pedicle, and is constructed from a fasciocutaneous island (epidermis, dermis, hypodermis and fascia) in the middle third of the leg [11, 16]. It can be turned distally to cover wounds of the distal third of the leg, ankle and foot. Its pedicle consists of the sural nerve, its nutritional artery (the superficial sural artery) and the small saphenous vein. The same flap can be based on a proximal pedicle and used to close defects around the knee.

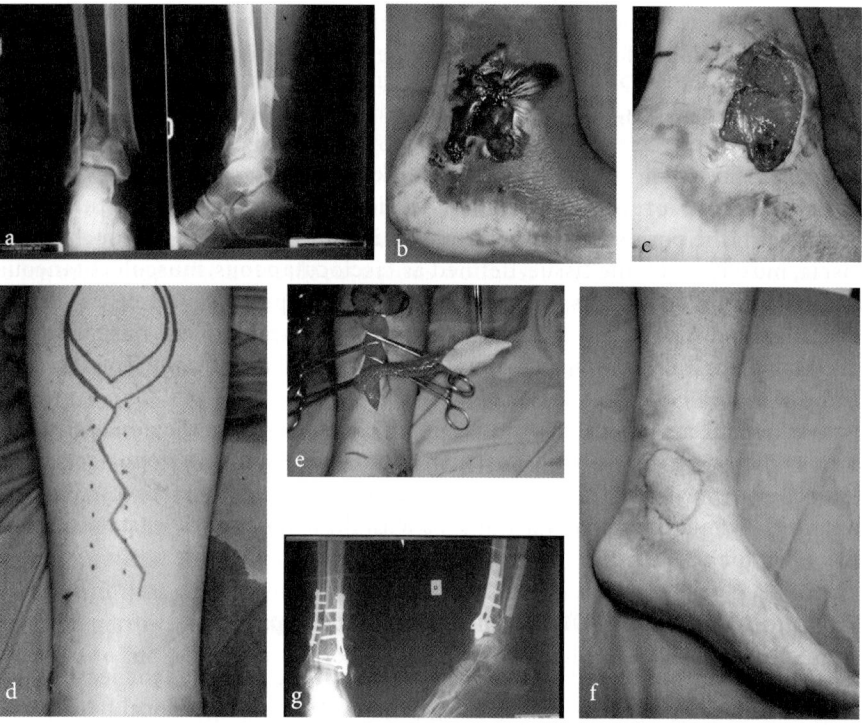

Fig. 1. a Pre-operative image of a tibial pilon fracture wound. **b** Soft tissue necrosis from high-energy trauma. **c** Extensive excision of all poorly vascularized necrotic tissue. **d** Planning of a fasciocutaneous sural island flap. **e** Preparation of the flap completed showing the arc of rotation. **f** Result one year later. **g** Internal fixation of the fracture

Anatomy

The sural nerve arises from the posterior tibial nerve, on average 6 cm behind the head of the fibula, and its main trunk has a constant course. Initially, it descends between the two heads of gastrocnemius, becoming increasingly superficial until it perforates the deep fascia at the junction of the superior and middle thirds of the leg. When it reaches the level of the lateral malleolus, the nerve branches terminally to the lateral side of the foot.

The superficial sural artery originates from the popliteal artery and passes distally between the two heads of gastrocnemius, joining the sural nerve after 2-3 cm, and sending a superficial cutaneous branch to the proximal third of the leg. It supplies the sural nerve during its subfascial course. After becoming superficial, it supplies cutaneous branches to the distal two-thirds of the leg.

There is a constant anastomosis with the septo-cutaneous branches of the peroneal artery at the level of the lateral malleolus in the tibio-fibular space. In 65% of cases the artery extends to the malleolar region, and in 35% it ends in a vascular network that supplies the distal third of the limb.

Positioning the Flap

A line is drawn on the skin along the entire subcutaneous course of the sural nerve, by tracing a vertical line between the two heads of gastrocnemius distal to the junction of the upper and middle thirds of the leg. The flap is incised from proximal to distal, sectioning proximally the artery, the sural nerve and the small saphenous vein. This neurovascular pedicle - which must include the subcutaneous and fascial tissue plus the superficial vein, when it exists - can be dissected down to a point 5 cm above the lateral malleolus, but no further, because distal to this pivot point there is a perforating branch from the peroneal artery that has a constant anastomosis with the superficial sural artery. This connection permits the formation of a distal pedicle flap with reverse vascularization from the peroneal artery.

Indications

The distal pedicle sural flap is used to fill soft tissue defects in the lower third of the leg, the ankle, the instep, the malleoli and the posterior calcaneal region.

Advantages

It has three significant advantages.

The operation is less complicated than a microsurgical procedure, requiring a simple preoperative Doppler evaluation and a short period for dissecting the flap.

Secondly, the main vascular axes of the leg are conserved when constructing this flap, enabling it to be utilised for tibial pilon fractures with severe vascular damage.

Finally, if the minor axis of the donor site is less than 4 cm, it can be closed primarily.

Disadvantages

The only disadvantage, which is relatively minor given the importance of the reconstruction, is the sacrifice of the sensation from the sural nerve. Following surgery all patients display differing degrees of paraesthesiae in the lateral portion of the foot, usually without more significant complications.

Extensor Digitorum Brevis Island Flap

This flap is generally used for defects in the proximal foot and malleolar regions, and is used less than the sural flap in complex fractures of the tibial pilon owing to its more limited arc of rotation and the smaller area of tissue that can be mobilised (Fig. 2) [17].

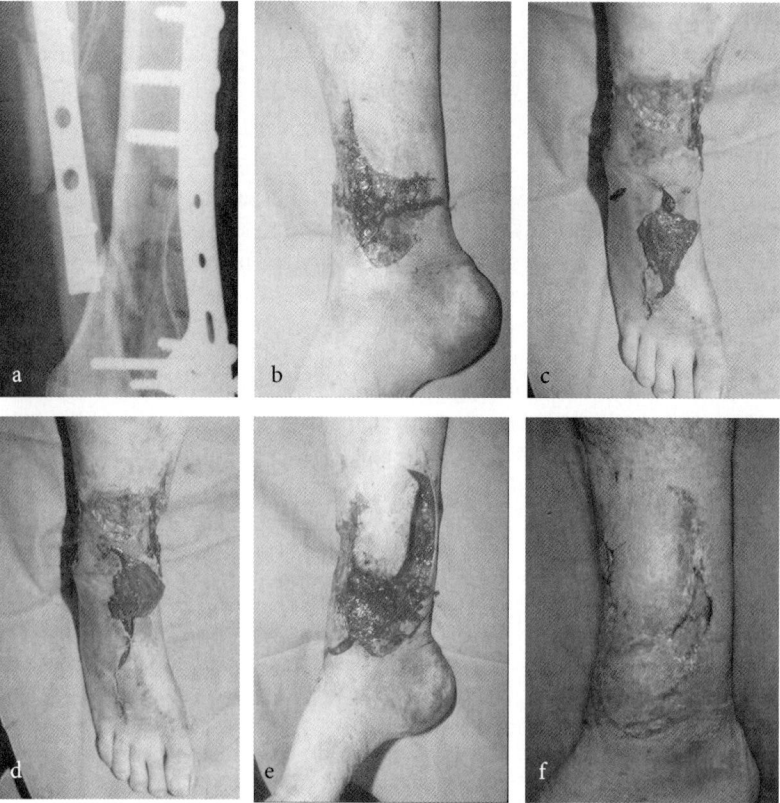

Fig. 2. a Fixation of a tibial pilon fracture. **b** Exposure of the tibial plate from necrosis of the overlying tissues. **c** Construction of an extensor digitorum brevis island flap. **d** Muscle tilted proximally before being transposed through a tunnel to the level of the defect. **e** Coverage of the wound with the foot muscle flap. **f** Result over time after placing a medium-thickness skin graft on the flap

Anatomy

Extensor digitorum brevis is wide and thin with a trapezoidal shape (4.5 cm wide and 6 cm long) and is located with extensor hallucis brevis on the dorsum of the foot, deep to the tendons of extensor digitorum longus and the branches of the superficial peroneal nerve and overlying the tarsal bones.

It originates from the lateral and superior portion of the calcaneus and splits into four tendons going distally and medially, the first of which is inserted into the base of the proximal phalanx of the hallux and the other three at the lateral edges of the tendon of extensor digitorum longus going to the second, third and fourth toes.

Although it has the function of extending the phalanges of the fully dorsiflexed foot and works synergistically with extensor digitorum longus, it can be sacrificed without significant loss of function.

Vascularization

The vascular supply to the muscle is provided by the lateral tarsal and arcuate arteries, branches of the dorsalis pedis, which penetrate proximally into the muscular belly.

Usually the lateral tarsal artery arises beneath the inferior extensor retinaculum and the arcuate artery 1-2 cm more distally.

The extensor digitorum flap deprives the dorsum of the foot of its main supply, the dorsalis pedis artery.

Part of the dorsum of the foot is also supplied by the terminal branches of the lateral calcaneal artery, which is a terminal branch of the peroneal artery, so the skin incision to approach this muscular flap must be medial to avoid depriving the dorsum of the foot of the vascular supply from the calcaneal vessels.

Innervation

The muscle is innervated by a branch of the deep peroneal nerve that penetrates the muscle proximally, in close contact with the vascular pedicle.

Indications

This muscular flap can be turned, proximally-based, both laterally and medially with a wide arc of rotation. Its size, approximately 5x7 cm, enables it to cover the lateral and medial malleoli, the distal insertion of the Achilles tendon, the calcaneus and the inferior third of the leg.

Because of its excellent blood supply, this flap is particularly indicated for infected wounds, as systemic antibiotics will reach the site of infection more easily and for soft tissue defects over a fracture, as the rich vascularization will stimulate periosteal activity and bone healing.

Operative Technique

The skin incision is at the back of the foot from the lateral malleolus to the base of the first metatarsal bone. The tendons of the extensor digitorum longus are displaced laterally, and the tendinous insertions of the muscle sectioned distally as closely as possible to their phalangeal attachments. The flap is lifted proximally and the two arterial pedicles identified, close to the extensor retinaculum. The dorsalis pedis artery is now ligated and sectioned distal to the origins of these branches to provide a free pedicle with two arteries, and veni comitantes. The donor area is closed by direct suture without the need for skin grafts.

Advantages

The extensor digitorum brevis flap presents various advantages:
-   it is easy technically;
-   the arterial pedicle is large calibre and has few anatomical variants;
-   it causes minimum morbidity to the donor region;
-   it is not very thick and adapts well to reconstruction of the lower limb;
-   it has a wide arc of rotation and will be useful for a variety of defects.

Posterior Fasciosubcutaneous Flap of the Leg

The posterior fasciocutaneous flap of the leg has more limited indications compared to the previous ones, but should not be neglected since it does not require the sacrifice of any major vascular axis.

Anatomy

Described by Marty and Montandon in 1984 on the basis of anatomical studies by Pearl and Johnson [18, 19], this flap is based on its own subcutaneous vascular plexus located between the loose and firm adipose tissue with a predominantly horizontal development.

Vascularization

The posterior fasciosubcutaneous flap of the leg receives its vascularization from 8 collateral branches of the posterior tibial artery at about 1 cm intervals which supply the subcutaneous tissue of the posterior aspect of the calf, each artery having an accompanying vein that ensures the venous return of the flap [20].

A second vascular supply is provided laterally by branches of the peroneal artery.

Another vascular supply is from the medial cutaneous sural artery which is a long subcutaneous branch of the medial sural artery going to the calcaneal tuberosity from the popliteal fossa.

This vascular model permits construction of a flap suitable for defects on the anterior surface of the leg, the heel and perimalleolar region and the posterior part of the foot.

Construction of the Flap

The special vascular characteristics of the subcutaneous tissue of the posterior surface of the leg allow a distal or "reverse" pedicle flap to be constructed. The size of the flap, and the possibility of turning it through 180°, permits coverage of areas otherwise difficult to reach.

Isolation of the distally-based flap must be preceded by meticulous planning. The upper edge must be placed 3-5 cm from the popliteal fossa, and distally dissection must stop 6-8 cm from the medial malleolus to conserve the septal branches of the posterior tibial artery. By making a median longitudinal incision limited to the dermis only, the dermoepidermal flaps can be raised exposing the subcutaneous tissue, which is incised around its perimeter according to the necessary dimensions, and comprises the muscular deep fascia that is attached to the subcutaneous adipose tissue with a few suture stitches. The small saphenous vein, which is sectioned and ligated, and the sural nerve should be conserved whenever possible, and are identified proximally. Dissection continues from proximal to distal along a subfascial plane up to 6-8 cm from the medial malleolus, where the flap can be turned or tilted to reach the receptor site. The flap is later covered with a thin skin graft, and the donor area is closed with direct sutures.

Advantages

The advantages of this flap are its easy execution, its versatility of use, its considerable size (20-25x12-15 cm) and the minimal aesthetic disturbance to the donor area. It also leaves the major vascular axes intact.

Disadvantages

This flap cannot be used when there are wounds or contusions in the distal two-thirds of the medial surface of the leg.

Other disadvantages are poor development of the subcutaneous tissue in some patients, and occasional marginal necrosis of the dermoepidermal flaps of the donor area.

Reconstruction of the Distal third of the Leg with Flaps from Remote Sites (Free Microsurgical Flaps)

Reconstruction with regional or local flaps is the method of choice, as it is the simplest solution and least costly for the patient. Unfortunately, it is not always practicable. When local damage is quite extensive, the creation of some flaps is prevented by wounds that affect their pedicles. The tissue defects may be so extensive that the local alternatives are insufficient.

The only solution in these cases is to bring in new tissue from regions undisturbed by trauma, which can be transferred as a free flap by microsurgical anastomosis [21, 22].

A microsurgical flap brings rich vascularization into the receptor region and increases the blood supply of the entire leg.

Indications for using Free Flaps

Microsurgical flaps are used for covering tibial pilon wounds in the following situations:

1. when there are no local solutions for covering extensive defects caused by wounds that affect the pedicles of potential local or regional flaps;
2. when the extent of the wound requires very large flaps not available locally;
3. as a "salvage" operation in the event of failure of local or regional flaps.

In all cases, anastomosis must be carried out remote from the traumatized area between anatomically healthy vessels not affected by the traumatic event.

There are different donor regions for such flaps, and choice depends on the site, dimensions and type of defect, the possible association of exposed bone or local infection, the presence of concomitant systemic illnesses such as diabetes or chronic renal insufficiency, the general condition of the tissues to be restored and the aesthetic and functional sequelae at the donor site.

Richly vascularized muscle flaps provide the highest stimulation to the fracture site, and adapt well to morphologically heterogeneous defects. They are particularly indicated for infection of the bone or surrounding soft tissues.

Contraindications for Using Free Flaps

It is not always possible to utilise a microvascular flap, as there are general and local contraindications.

General contraindications comprise all the pathology that can negatively affect the integrity of small-calibre vessels and consequently vascular micro-anastomoses, such as atherosclerosis, progressive diabetes, hypertension, Raynaud's Disease, etc. The probability of surgical success in these conditions is significantly reduced, to the extent that the procedure is contra-indicated.

Local damage to the receptor vessels may also prevent the use of this technique.

Local inflammation or bacterial infection, especially if chronic, may cause fibrosis and loss of vessel elasticity that will result in greater difficulty for the anastomosis. Evaluation of the patency of the receptor vessels and the global vascularization of the leg by angiography is advisable prior to executing a free flap, since one of the main arterial trunks must receive the microanastomosis.

In emergency, the integrity of the receptor vessels must be evaluated directly in the operating theatre, ascertaining also the precise function of the other vascular axes. It is also important to observe any vascular changes (cyanosis, pallor of the limb) secondary to clamping the vein and artery that are to be used for end to end anastomosis.

Advantages

There are several advantages of using microvascular flaps:
- only one operation may be required;
- the flap to be used can be chosen for its morphological characteristics: size, thickness, colour, innervation, presence of hair and the possibility of being able also to include bone tissue and tendons;
- when using free flaps, there is a significant reduction in the time for immobilisation compared to classic methods, such as the cross-leg technique, or reconstruction over several operations;
- there should be a global improvement in the perfusion of the lower limb.

Disadvantages

- the operation and anaesthetic time is long, normally 4-8 hours. The length of the operation depends on the experience of the surgeon and how well the team work together; it can be shortened by using two surgical teams simultaneously, and by the type of flap used, the dissection of which may be more or less difficult;
- there is the risk of vascular thrombosis and other complications.

There are three important stages that lead to microvascular flap success:

Preoperative Evaluation of the Receptor Region

This must be as accurate as possible and aim at identifying uninjured vessels suitable for microvascular anastomosis.

In the acute phase, it is not easy to define the area of damage and then identify the healthy structures. Helpful management includes early antibiotic treatment, surgical cleansing of the devitalised tissues, repeated additional debridement as required to prepare the wound to receive a free flap, which should be performed, if possible, within two weeks of the trauma.

Pedicle Suture

During pedicle suture, we recommend suturing the venous anastomosis first and then the arterial anastomosis, to reduce blood loss and to prevent venous stagnation in the flap.

Also, it is better to avoid clamping the vessels again after the artery has been sutured to reduce the risk of thrombosis.

An end to end anastomosis is generally preferred, but end to side anastomosis is often used in the leg, owing to the type of vessels and the smaller number available.

Flaps with long pedicles allow anastomosis to be performed with remote and therefore safe receptor vessels.

Postoperative Monitoring

When applying dressings, circumferential bandages must be avoided to minimise the risk of compressing the flap pedicle. Monitoring is done by direct observation of the flap vitality and by checking the patient's general status, such as heart rate and arterial pressure, body temperature, diuresis, haematocrit and coagulation parameters.

Complications

These can be general or local.

General complications can be related to the duration of anaesthesia, extended operating time and postural factors causing an increase in venous stasis, followed by deep vein thrombosis and consequent pulmonary thromboembolism.

Local complications are vascular and are generally caused by vasospasm or vasal thrombosis.

Vasospasm is solely a functional problem and treatment is medical, but surgical inspection of the anastomosis is necessary in the case of arterial or venous thrombosis.

Free muscular Flaps

They consist of a muscle that is completely severed from its osteotendinous attachments and transferred with its main pedicle to a remote receptor region where microvascular anastomosis is performed [23].

Latissimus Dorsi Free Flap

Anatomy

The latissimus dorsi is fan-shaped, wide and relatively thin. Three of its borders can be defined by its bony attachments. It originates medially from the last thoracic and lumbosacral vertebrae, and distally from the medial half of the iliac crest, and is inserted into the proximal third of the humerus through a wide, thin tendon. The superior edge passes in an arc close to the inferior corner of the scapula, and the lateral edge can be palpated in all patients if the muscle is contracted.

Vascularization

The main pedicle is made up of the thoracodorsal artery, one of the two branches of the subscapular artery, which arises from the third part of the axillary artery. The subscapular artery gives off the circumflex scapular artery, which traverses the triangular space, and ends by dividing into the artery to serratus anterior and the thoracodorsal artery, which continues distally as the dominant pedicle supplying latissimus dorsi.

Entry of the thoracodorsal artery into the muscle is located on average about 7-8 cm from the origin of the scapular artery [24].

Innervation

The muscle is innervated by the thoracodorsal nerve, a branch of the posterior cord of the brachial plexus, behind the axillary artery and vein, and with the artery and vein constitutes the flap's pedicle [25].

Indications

The latissimus dorsi free flap is indicated for the elective repair of extensive soft tissue loss, especially in areas subject to considerable mechanical stress (Fig. 3) [26, 27].

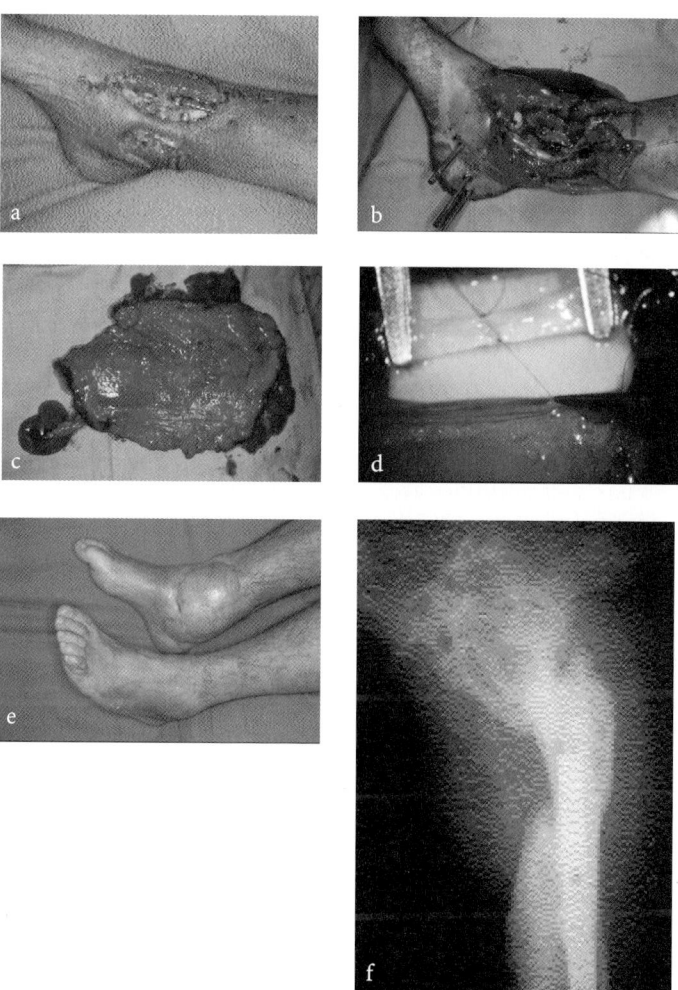

Fig. 3. a Pre-operative image of extensive loss of skin and bone loss complicated by infection. **b** Thorough debridement of all necrotic tissues, removal of implanted metal and application of an external fixator. **c** Construction of a free latissimus dorsi flap sufficient to salvage the distal extremity of the leg and foot. **d** Microsurgical suture of the vascular pedicle. **e** Result two years after the trauma. **f** The result after two years is satisfactory regarding the soft tissue reconstruction, but the choice of the method of synthesis in this open fracture, complicated by infection, have led to spontaneous arthrodesis of the tibiotarsal joint. In this case, poor planning of the primary surgery produced disappointing functional results

Operative Technique

The patient is placed in the lateral recumbent position for dissecting the flap. The skin and subcutaneous tissue are incised from the posterior axillary wall along the tenth rib so as to permit wide exposure. The superior, posterior, inferior and anterior margins of the muscle are identified, after which the deep plane is developed, starting from the lateral portions of the muscle and proceeding medially. The serratus anterior muscle is left with the intercostal muscles and remains adherent to the thoracic wall. Care is required in dissecting the deep plane in the axilla to avoid damaging the neurovascular pedicle, which is freed up to its origin. It is necessary to ligate the branch leading to the serratus anterior muscle.

When the pedicle is identified, the muscle is sectioned along its edges with careful haemostasis.

It is now possible to section the pedicle, having identified its structures, and make the microvascular anastomoses.

Advantages

Dissection is quick and easy, and safe enough by virtue of the absence of anatomical vascular changes at the pedicle level. It has a good length and the vessels that form it have a wide calibre.

The flap has a large surface area, and produces an excellent result. There are no significant functional sequelae after this muscle has been removed.

Disadvantages

The flap remains quite thick even after some time, despite the usual atrophy from denervation. Additional plastic procedures may be required. The scar at the donor site often remains highly visible.

Serratus Anterior Flap

This flap is formed from just the last three digitations of serratus anterior to prevent the onset of winged scapula, which would occur if its first digitations were sacrificed.

Anatomy

The muscle originates from the external surface and superior edge of the first 8-9 ribs and inserts into the vertebral edge of the scapula. It has a wide, flat shape and consists of several digitations.

Vascularization

The first 4-5 superior digitations are supplied by the thoracolateral artery, and the inferior digitations by the thoracodorsal artery, which together with the comitant veins constitutes the vascular pedicle of the flap.

Innervation

The nerve to serratus anterior is a direct branch of the anterior primary rami of the 5th, 6th and 7th cervical nerve roots, and runs along the anterior margin of the muscle, joining the branch of the thoracodorsal artery at the level of the 6th digitation, and during its course supplies branches to each digitation.

Indications

Since it is a medium-sized muscular flap, it is indicated for all complex soft tissue loss for which local or rotated fasciocutaneous flaps would not be sufficient and a latissimus dorsi flap would be too large.

Operative Technique

The patient is placed in a lateral recumbent position and the skin incision follows the anterior border of latissimus dorsi on the lateral thoracic wall from the posterior axillary fold.

The anterior border of latissimus dorsi is exposed, and the plane between this muscle dorsally and the serratus anterior developed in a dorsal direction. The thoracodorsal neurovascular bundle is identified during this manoeuvre.

Careful dissection of the vessels identifies 1 or 2 branches to serratus anterior, generally from the thoracodorsal vessel at the level of the 6th rib, supplying the most distal muscle bellies.

The last three thoracic digitations are freed from the thoracic wall by sectioning their attachments to the ribs. The latissimus dorsi vascular branch is ligated and having sectioned the muscle from its scapular attachment, the flap can be removed with its pedicle.

Advantages

The flap has a long vascular pedicle that is therefore adaptable to various clinical situations.

Because of the common origins of the serratus anterior and latissimus dorsi flap pedicles, it is possible to use these flaps "combined".

Disadvantages

The most important disadvantage may derive from an iatrogenic error during dissection and it consists of the possibility of the onset of the winged scapula phenomenon if the innervation of the first muscular digitations is not preserved.

Gracilis Flap

Anatomy

The gracilis [8] is a long ribbon-like muscle on the medial face of the thigh originating from the anterior face of the ischium and inferior pubic ramus near the symphysis, and then goes downwards vertically inserting at the level of the tibial tuberosity together with the sartorius and semitendinous muscles with which it forms the pes anserinus tendon [23].

Vascularization

The muscle has a main pedicle and at least two secondary pedicles. The former is a branch of the medial femoral circumflex artery, a branch of the profunda femoris artery, with its concomitant veins, and enters the muscle about 10 cm below the pubic symphysis [21].

The secondary pedicles arise from the superficial femoral artery.

Innervation

Gracilis is innervated by the obturator nerve that runs between adductor longus and adductor brevis in the thigh. It divides into motor and sensory branches near the main vascular pedicle. The motor nerve enters the muscle and splits into two branches; the sensory nerve, which has a vertical downward course, perforates the muscle in its central portion and innervates the overlying skin.

Indications

Gracilis can be used as a local, rotated flap for loss of tissue in the groin, thigh, genitals and perineum.

It is indicated as a free flap particularly when there are rectangular areas of tissue loss, for which the muscle is an ideal shape.

Operative Procedure

The patient is positioned supine with the thigh abducted and the knee flexed.

The anterior border of gracilis corresponds to a line between the posterior border of the tendon of adductor longus and the pubic tubercle.

The skin incision down to the deep fascia follows this line over the medial surface of the thigh. The most important vessels are located 8 cm from the pubic tubercle. The fascia is sectioned to locate the interval between adductor longus and gracilis. Having retracted the adductor longus laterally, the vascular pedicle and anterior branch of the obturator nerve can be identified.

The muscle is located distally between sartorius and semimembranosus. Collateral branches of the femoral vessels (secondary pedicles) penetrate the muscle at this level and should be ligated. The distal portion of the muscle is detached, followed by the proximal portion, sectioning the main pedicle near its origin so that it is as long as possible.

Advantages

The vascular pedicle is constant, as is its course and entry point into the muscle. The vessels forming the pedicle have adequate calibre for microsurgical sutures.

The donor site can be closed directly and the linear scar on the medial surface of the thigh does not cause aesthetic problems.

Sacrifice of the gracilis does not produce a functional deficiency.

Disadvantages

The main disadvantage is the short length of the vascular pedicle, usually less than 5 cm.

Free Fasciocutaneous Flaps

Radial Forearm Flap or Chinese Flap

This is a fasciocutaneous flap taken from the volar surface of the forearm (radial side) in its distal third [28].

Anatomy and Vascularization

The vascular pedicle is provided by the radial artery and its comitant veins. This vessel of the distal third of the forearm is relatively superficial and is located near the flexion fold of the wrist. In the hand, it reaches the palmar vascular plane where anastomosis with the ulnar artery is constant, whether by direct arcuate anastomosis or through collaterals.

The presence of the distal anastomosis allows this area to be taken as a free flap.

In the distal part of its route, the radial artery gives off collateral branches in constant formation that supply the skin of the forearm.

Operative Technique

It is necessary to check the patency of the two arterial axes, radial and ulnar, prior to constructing the Chinese flap. Although it may generally be sufficient to do Allen's test, at times an angiographic investigation may be necessary. Allen's test evaluates whether sacrifice of the radial artery compromises the vascularization of the hand.

The operation starts by drawing the radial axis on the skin, from the fold of the elbow right to the groove of the wrist. The margins of the flap are then drawn with the axis corresponding to the cutaneous projection of the radial artery.

Dissection begins with identification of the flap pedicle at the proximal border, where the artery and comitant veins are separately dissected and ligated.

The skin incision is then performed down to the deep fascia, to include the entire circumference of the island flap.

The lateral cutaneous nerve of the forearm is usually sectioned at the point where it enters the proximal border of the flap. In contrast, the sensory superficial cutaneous branch of the radial nerve must be preserved.

After the ulnar and radial borders of the flap have been raised, it remains attached to the bone via the deep intermuscular septum. This is now sectioned and all branches of the radial artery to adjacent muscles are ligated.

Excision of the flap is completed by dissecting the radial pedicle down to the most distal wrist flexion crease, where it is ligated and incised.

Finally the donor region is covered with thin split skin grafts.

Advantages

There are many advantages to this technique. The anatomy of the vascular pedicle is constant with an absence of anatomical variants. It is a reliable flap that

Short and Long Term Results

Short and Long Term Results of Treatment

B. Magnan, E. Facci, M. Veronese, N. Rossi, P. Bartolozzi

The long term prognosis of tibial pilon fractures depends on the type of fracture and is directly correlated to the fracture classification, as suggested by several authors [1-5].

The incidence of poor results increases with the severity of the fracture. Following Ruedi and Allgower's classification [3], McFerran and colleagues in 1992 [6] and Teeny and Wiss in 1993 [7] indicated a percentage of complications of around 30% for Types I and II, and between 42% and 70% for Type III. This percentage would today be considered rather pessimistic for Type I, but remains realistic for Type III.

The poor results of tibial pilon fractures can be considered *short-term* and *long-term* [8-10]. The former includes skin breakdown and early infection with an incidence of approximately 20%. Long term complications are osteitis (17%), malunion (42%), nonunion (18%), joint stiffness (27%) and post-traumatic arthrosis, which is the most frequent complication with an incidence of more than 50%.

Considering the treatment of these complications, for *osteitis*, the treatment of choice is not specific for tibial pilon fractures and consists of resection of the infected segment associated with reconstructive surgery, which may require bone transport, possibly associated with plastic surgery. Traditional measures such as debridement, lavage and antibiotic treatment, possibly associated with hyperbaric oxygen treatment can still be implemented.

Malunion may be a varus or valgus deformity, rotational defect, length discrepancy, or malposition of the malleoli or portions of the tibial plafond. To prevent articular degeneration, treatment of such problems must be early (within a year), and ideally before the onset of articular degeneration. *Intra-articular reconstructive surgery* may be achieved by osteotomies of the malleoli, or

Clinica Ortopedica e Traumatologica, Università degli Studi di Verona

the tibial platfond as suggested by Lelièvre in 1981, or by fibula osteotomy generally with lengthening. Alternatively, *extra-articular reconstructive surgery* can be performed with tibial or fibular osteotomies followed by progressive callus distraction of an articulated external fixator following the hemicallotasis technique.

In 1979, Rosemayer defined the indications for extra-articular osteotomy as a varus deformity >6° or valgus >12°, whereas, in 1989, Kristensen recommended its use for varus or -valgus deformities >15°.

For *nonunion*, non-invasive treatment can be used, such as extracorporeal shock waves or pulsed electromagnetic fields, but secondary surgery is frequently required to achieve stable internal fixation with compression often including decortication and bone graft, or arthrodesis when distal areas are involved or when there is articular involvement.

Joint stiffness must be treated as early as possible, with procedures such as cheilectomy, debridement and chondral abrasion, by arthrotomy or arthroscopy. Other techniques are interposition arthroplasty or arthrodiatasis, which is a surgical technique suggested by Renzi Brivio and Aldegheri in 1986, in which cheilectomy, synovectomy and debridement are performed with an open procedure, and an articulated external fixator applied with 4-5 mm of distraction. Intense early mobilisation is specified, and total treatment time lasts about 3 months.

The original biological hypothesis for this methodology was to permit the formation of fibrocartilage able to support weight-bearing. In 1999 van Roermund presented arthrodiatasis as a technique able to provide a stimulus for the repair of degenerated articular cartilage, while reducing mechanical stresses and maintaining the cyclical pressure of the intra-articular fluid.

In the original proposal, arthrodiatasis was used in 12 cases with a follow-up today of more than 18 years. It was reviewed more recently by van Roermund and colleagues in 1999 and in 2002 [11], and by Amendola in 2002, for a total of 50 cases, with a follow-up ranging from 1 to 7 years.

In a review published in 1989 by Nogarin and colleagues [12], the results of this surgical technique were defined as "modest on the radiographic level, but more encouraging on the functional level and good regarding the pain symptoms". When analysing the cases reviewed after a period of about 20 years, an asymptomatic ankylosis was obtained with the tibiotarsal joint in a good position, but inevitably a functional result insufficient in terms of movement.

In treating *advanced post-traumatic arthrosis*, there is an interesting alternative between *arthrodesis* and *arthroprosthesis*. Both procedures have the same indications: persistent pain, articular stiffness, significant deformity and instability.

Until now, arthrodesis was considered the correct treatment for younger patients with greater functional demands, reserving use of a prosthesis for older patients. Today, however, an artificial ankle joint is more in demand also for younger patients who have post-traumatic pathology and greater functional requirements, and who tolerate the loss of ankle function poorly. Current experience of tibiotarsal prosthetic implants is that the joint tends towards asymptomatic ankylosis rather than painful instability, as is often found in the hip or knee.

What is important in pre-operative planning is assessment of the function of the subtalar and midtarsal joints, because should they also be involved, as often occurs in post-traumatic cases, retaining the function of the ankle joint is even more critical.

Axial deviation or non union may lastly be technical complications of a prosthetic implant.

More than 30 *tibiotarsal arthrodesis techniques* have been described. There follows a description of the 5 most popular methods, with which the authors have had personal experience.

An *arthrotomy* by an anteromedial or anterolateral approach, resection of any medial and lateral osteophyte impingements and joint surfaces, and internal fixation with 2 cannulated screws by a lateral approach from the talus and tibia or a medial and lateral proximo-distal approach.

Transperoneal arthrotomy proposed by Horvitz in 1942, renewed by Adams in 1948 and publicised in the 1990s by Malerba [13]. The fibula is resected and tilted downwards while maintaining the distal ligamentous anchorage. Excision of the joint surfaces is performed, with a brace as Malerba suggests, and then the fibia is again reattached with 2 cannulated screws in the tibial and talar regions.

Arthrodesis by arthroscopy may be used where there is no length discrepancy to be corrected (Morgan 1991, Myerson and Qill 1991).

The *mini-arthrotomy technique* is derived from the arthroscopy technique and it specifies medial and lateral mini-incisions, according to Gallie's technique continued by Myerson, and the use of two cylindrical corticocancellous bone grafts taken from the iliac crest and stabilised with braces or screws.

Finally, arthrodesis with *external fixation* under compression is used in special situations, when there are infections, musculocutaneous complications or in association with a proximal bone transport.

There are also various models that have been proposed over the years in the case of *tibiotarsal arthroprosthesis*: from the historical St. George-Bucholz, Smith, Pipino-Calderale, Mayo and TPR to the more modern LCS, Agilità, Assenzio, Hintegra and STAR. Present-day arthroprosthesis is made up of three elements. It is congruent, unconstrained and has a mobile meniscus.

The corrective potential of the prosthetic implant with axial screws is limited to between 5° and 10°, even if some authors believe corrections are possible up to 20°. Higher values should lead to consideration of axial correction before proceeding with the prosthetic implant, or whether the two procedures can be performed at the same time.

Finally, it is reasonable to consider the need for specific tibial components before treating particular cases.

In conclusion, poor results of tibial pilon fractures have an incidence from 30% to 70%, and correlate more with the type of fracture than the method of treatment. A severe degenerative arthropathy may start as a long-term complication in more than 50% of cases. This outcome should no longer be treated with "conservative" surgery, which has led to disappointing results.

Arthrodesis and arthroprosthesis are the two current alternatives. The former provides good results in 80-90% of cases; it requires experience and good surgical technique. The indication for arthroprosthesis has today has been extended to younger patients, but its effectiveness tends to deteriorate over time, and insertion can be technically difficult in post-traumatic cases, so that at times custom prostheses may be necessary.

Treatment of malunion is useful if performed at an early stage, i.e. within one year.

Soft tissue infection and complications radically affect the choice of treatment.

References

1. Lauge–Hansen N (1953) Fractures of the ankle V: pronation–dorsiflection fractures. Arch Surg 67:813
2. Gay R, Evrard J (1963) Les fractures recentes du pilon tibial chez l'adulte. Rev Chir Orthop 49:397
3. Ruedi T, Allgower M (1979) The operative treatment of intra-articular fractures of the lower end of the tibia. Clin Orthop Rel Res 138:105-110
4. Vives P, Hourlier H, De Lastang M et al (1984) 84 fractures of the lower end of the tibia in adults. Attempt at a classification. Rev Chir Orthop Reparatrice Appar Mot 70(2):129-139
5. Müller ME, Nazarian S, Koch P et al (1990) Classification of the fractures of the long bones. Springer, Berlin Heidelberg New York
6. Mc Ferran MA, Smith SW, Boulas J, Schwartz HS (1992) Complications encountered in the treatment of pilon fractures. J Orthop Traumat 6(2):195-200
7. Teeny SM, Wiss DA (1993) Open reduction and internal fixation of tibial plafond fractures: variables contributing to poor results and complications. Clin Orthop Rel Res 292:108-117
8. Ceccarelli F, Girolami M, Bertelli R, Giannini S (1992) Vizi di consolidazione nelle fratture di tibio-tarsica. Progressi in medicina e chirurgia del piede, Vol.1: fratture della tibio-tarsica. Aulo Gaggi, Milano
9. Ruedi T, Allgower M (1983) Die Frakturen des Pilon Tibial. Unfallheilkunde 86:259-261
10. Thordarson DB (2000) Complications after treatment of tibial pilon fractures: prevention and management strategies. J Am Acad Orthop Surg 8(4):253-265
11. Van Roermund P (2002) Joint distraction as an alternative for treatment of osteoarthritis. Proceedings of the 32nd Annual Meeting of the AOFAS, Dallas
12. Nogarin L, Magnan B, Brigantini A et al (1989) Fratture recenti ed inveterate del collo del piede trattate con FEA. Chir del piede 13:311-20
13. Malerba F, De Marchi F (1992) Artrodesi della tibio-tarsica negli esiti di fratture malleolari. Progressi in medicina e chirurgia del piede, Vol.1: fratture della tibio-tarsica. Aulo Gaggi, Milano

Consensus

At the end of the conference proceedings a consensus on the methods and options for treating the more severe closed and open tibial pilon fractures (Group C3 according to the AO classification) was reached and they are outlined hereunder in Tables 1, 2, 3 and 4.

Table 1. Closed tibial pilon fractures

Type of fracture	Treatment options	
Type C1 fracture	Internal fixation	External fixation with minimal internal fixation in case of metaphyseal extension
Type C2 fracture	External fixation with minimal internal fixation	Internal fixation
Type C 3 fracture	External fixation with minimal internal fixation	Temporary external fixation followed by internal fixation

Table 2. Type 1 open fractures according to Anderson-Gustilo

Type of fracture	Treatment options	
Type C1 fracture	Internal fixation	External fixation with minimal internal fixation in case of metaphyseal extension
Type C2 fracture	External fixation with minimal internal fixation	Internal fixation
Type C3 fracture	External fixation with minimal internal fixation	Temporary external fixation followed by internal fixation

Table 3. Type 2, 3A and 3B open fractures according to Anderson-Gustilo

Type of fracture	Treatment options
Type C1 fracture	External fixation with minimal internal fixation
Type C2 fracture	External fixation with minimal internal fixation
Type C3 fracture	External fixation with/without minimal internal fixation

Table 4. Type 3C open fractures according to Anderson-Gustilo

Type of fracture	Treatment options	
Type C1 fracture	External fixation with minimal internal fixation	Amputation
Type C 2 fracture	fracture External fixation with minimal internal fixation	Amputation
Type C 3 fracture	fracture External fixation with/without minimal internal fixation	Amputation

Subject Index